The Blue Zone Blueprint

Unlocking the Secrets to a Longer, Healthier Life

By
Alex Sterling

The Blue Zone Blueprint

Unlocking the Secrets to a Longer, Healthier Life

Table of Contents

Introduction

We're all in search of the secret to a long, healthy, and fulfilling life. Yet, the answers are often deceptively simple and within reach for anyone willing to make small but impactful changes. Welcome to a journey that transcends the boundaries of age, genetics, and geography, transcending traditional views of health and wellness. This book aims to empower you with actionable strategies drawn from the lives of the world's longest-lived and healthiest communities, known as Blue Zones. It's about blending scientific insights with anecdotal wisdom to pave a personalized path towards longevity and quality of life.

Imagine communities where people not only live longer but also stay vital and avoid many of the chronic diseases plaguing modern society. These Blue Zones are unique regions where individuals live significantly longer, happier lives than the average person. The power of community, a sense of purpose, and balanced living plays a pivotal role in their extraordinary health and longevity. By examining their daily habits, dietary choices, and social structures, we can glean valuable lessons that are both practical and inspirational.

This isn't merely a theoretical compilation but a practical guide designed to be your companion in transforming your life. Each chapter delves into the essential elements that contribute to longevity, supported by evidence-based research and enriched with motivational stories that can propel you to take meaningful action. While science sets the stage, it's the real-life applications that will make all the difference in your journey.

Our first step together will be uncovering the magic of the Blue Zones. These aren't just geographical locations; they are a goldmine of wisdom that has defied aging and promoted health through simple but profound lifestyle choices. Understanding why these zones matter is crucial as they provide a template anyone can adapt, irrespective of where they live. In doing so, you will discover not just nutritional guidelines or exercise tips, but a holistic lifestyle model that encompasses social connections, purpose, spirituality, and well-being.

Moreover, we'll explore the undeniable impact of a supportive community. Having a strong network of friends and family isn't just comforting; it's a lifesaving resource. Studies consistently show that people with robust social ties have lower risks of chronic illnesses. So, it's high time we appreciate the village that surrounds us and find ways to foster it for our benefit.

Nutrition is another cornerstone of longevity, often shrouded in myths and misleading information. The Blue Zones diet shuns extremes and embraces moderation, promoting plant-based, whole food choices that are both delicious and nourishing. It's not merely about what we eat, but how we eat that matters. Incorporating traditional recipes and dietary habits from these regions can seamlessly blend joy and health together.

Physical movement shouldn't be confined to a gym routine. Blue Zones inhabitants engage in natural, daily activities that keep their bodies in perpetual motion. These aren't structured exercises but lifestyle movements such as gardening, walking, and even routine chores, all contributing to their physical and mental well-being. Through this book, you'll learn to weave movement into your everyday life, making fitness a joyful part of your routine.

Having a clear sense of purpose, or "ikigai," as it's called in Okinawa, has profound effects on longevity and happiness. Identifying and nurturing something that gets you out of bed in the morning can significantly boost your overall well-being. Whether it's a hobby, a career, or a cause, finding your personal ikigai can serve as a powerful motivator to lead a longer, more fulfilling life.

It's a fast-paced world, and stress seems almost inescapable. Yet, Blue Zones communities excel at managing it through relaxation techniques, spirituality, and the gift of downtime. Learning how to incorporate these practices into your daily routine can create a buffer against the detrimental effects of chronic stress and improve your quality of life.

Your living environment also has a profound impact on your health. Small changes in your surroundings can promote sustainable living and transform your home into a personal Blue Zone. From decluttering to creating restful spaces, every little tweak counts towards building an environment that nurtures longevity.

Faith and spirituality are woven into the fabric of Blue Zones' daily life. Engaging in regular spiritual practices, whether through organized religion or personal rituals, has been shown to enhance emotional well-being and provide a soothing sense of purpose. It's about finding what aligns with your beliefs and making it a steadfast part of your routine.

Quality sleep is not just a luxury but a necessity. The habits and environment conducive to restorative sleep are pillars of health in Blue Zones. Understanding these can help you adjust your routines and environment to secure the rest your body and mind crave.

Each chapter of this book serves as both a lesson and a guide, generously sprinkled with practical tips and motivational stories from Blue Zones. From developing positive daily habits to avoiding harmful behaviors, you'll find pathways to incorporate these life-enhancing changes into your lifestyle. Through establishing routines and breaking free from damaging practices, you can set a course toward a healthier, more fulfilling life.

Finally, we're living in an age where scientific advancements continuously unearth new insights into longevity. Bridging the gap between age-old wisdom and modern science is not only enlightening but essential for crafting a comprehensive approach to health. This book dives into existing research and future directions in longevity science, offering you a well-rounded understanding of what's possible.

By the end of our journey together, you'll have a blueprint for transforming your life. Whether it's actionable tips, real-life success stories, or a tailored plan for your unique needs, you'll find yourself equipped to forge a path toward longevity and enriched quality of life. Your transformation awaits, and it promises not just extra years but better years.

So, let's embark on this journey together, blending wisdom with action, and creating a life that's not just longer, but more vibrant and fulfilling. This introduction is merely the beginning, a gateway to a world of possibilities waiting to be explored and embraced.

Chapter 1:
Discovering the Blue Zones

Venturing into the concept of Blue Zones is like uncovering a treasure map to longevity. These distinct geographical areas, such as Okinawa in Japan and Sardinia in Italy, showcase populations that not only live longer but also enjoy healthier and more vibrant lives. Understanding what makes these zones unique gives us practical insights into how we might emulate their success. It's not just about diet or exercise; it's a holistic approach that includes strong community ties, purposeful living, and natural movement. As we dive deeper into the history and significance of Blue Zones, we'll unearth strategies that are both simple and profound, paving the way for a healthier and longer life tailored to our unique circumstances.

What Are Blue Zones?

Blue Zones are unique regions around the world where people live significantly longer and healthier lives compared to the global average. These areas have become the gold standard for longevity research and have attracted the attention of scientists, researchers, and health enthusiasts. Essentially, Blue Zones serve as living laboratories that offer critical insights into the secrets of a long, fulfilling life.

The term "Blue Zones" originates from the work of demographers and researchers who circled these areas on maps with blue ink. Identified through data-driven approaches and meticulous field research, these zones include Okinawa in Japan, Sardinia in Italy, Ikaria in

Greece, Nicoya Peninsula in Costa Rica, and Loma Linda in California. Each of these places boasts high numbers of centenarians—people who live to be 100 years or older. But longevity isn't simply about adding years to your life; it's about adding life to your years.

You might wonder what sets Blue Zones apart from the rest of the world. The answer lies in a harmonious blend of genetics, lifestyle choices, and social structures. People in these regions naturally integrate healthy habits into their daily routines, almost effortlessly. They don't necessarily aim to live longer; their environments, cultures, and practices inherently promote longevity. Imagine living in a place where the default activities encourage better health.

One of the most striking features of Blue Zones is their diet. Although there's variation depending on geography and culture, a predominantly plant-based diet unites these regions. Whole foods, minimal processed foods, and balanced nutrition form the crux of their eating habits. You won't find large quantities of meat or sugary snacks. Instead, you'll see lots of vegetables, fruits, grains, and legumes. For instance, Okinawans are known for their consumption of sweet potatoes and soy products. This emphasis on nutrient-dense, natural foods plays a crucial role in their sustained good health.

Another shared characteristic is regular physical activity, but not in the way you might think. Gym sessions or running marathons aren't common in Blue Zones. Instead, people engage in low-intensity, consistent physical activities like walking, gardening, or dancing. These activities are woven into the fabric of their daily lives. The results? Remarkable health benefits, better mobility in old age, and high energy levels throughout life.

You can't talk about Blue Zones without mentioning the power of community and social connections. These regions place a high value on family, friendships, and social engagement. For example, in Sardinia, multi-generational living is common, and elderly family members are well-integrated into social activities. This builds strong support systems and offers regular opportunities for emotional connection. The sense of belonging and community significantly contributes to mental well-being and overall happiness.

Furthermore, Blue Zone residents usually have a strong sense of purpose—referred to as "ikigai" in Okinawa or "plan de vida" in Nicoya. This purpose often comes from their role within the community, work they find meaningful, or a passion that drives them daily. Having a sense of purpose is linked to lower stress levels and better mental health, thereby contributing to a longer lifespan.

Stress management is yet another critical element. Unlike the high-pressure environments many of us find ourselves in, the inhabitants of Blue Zones have mastered the art of relaxation and taking time for themselves. Whether it's through prayer, meditation, or simply spending time in nature, they incorporate regular relaxation techniques into their routines. This helps them maintain lower stress levels, which in turn reduces the risk of chronic diseases like heart disease and diabetes.

The environments in Blue Zones also play a part. These places often enjoy favorable climates, which encourage outdoor activities and social gatherings. Communities are designed in such a way that promotes interaction and physical activity. For instance, many towns and villages have centralized gathering spots where community events are held. Beaches, hills, and walking paths are common—everything seems set up to facilitate a healthy lifestyle.

Faith and spirituality also form an essential part of life in Blue Zones. It's not necessarily about religion, but rather a deeper connection to something greater than oneself. This sense of spirituality offers comfort, reduces stress, and fosters a sense of belonging. Regular practices, whether attending church services or community gatherings, strengthen social bonds and provide emotional support, essential elements for a healthy life.

Sleep is another aspect that tops the lists of healthy habits in Blue Zones. People in these areas prioritize rest and ensure they get quality sleep. Unlike the hustle culture prevalent in many parts of the world, taking naps and going to bed early is normalized. Good sleep hygiene is critical for mental health, cognitive function, and physical recovery, all of which contribute to longevity.

But perhaps one of the most crucial ingredients in the Blue Zones recipe for a long life is their cultural approach to health. Health and well-being are not afterthoughts, nor are they viewed as separate from daily life. Instead, they are part and parcel of every decision, every meal, and every interaction. This cultural embedding of health priorities makes sticking to beneficial habits second nature to the residents.

The idea of creating your own Blue Zone might seem daunting, but it's more achievable than you think. Simple changes—like fostering closer relationships, eating more plant-based foods, incorporating regular physical activity, and finding your purpose—can significantly improve your chances of living a long, healthy life. The Blue Zones offer us a glimpse into what a life well-lived looks like, inviting us to make tangible changes to our own lives.

Ultimately, understanding what Blue Zones are offers invaluable lessons on how to live longer and better. The magic isn't in a single superfood or an exotic exercise regimen but in the holistic way of life. It's a call to re-evaluate and redesign our lives to embody balance, purpose, and community. The journey to longevity doesn't have a fixed start or end; it's about incorporating sustainable practices that align with the core principles observed in Blue Zones. So, what's stopping you from creating your own Blue Zone right where you are?

The History of Blue Zones Research

As we dive into the history of Blue Zones research, it's fascinating to uncover how it all began and evolved. Researchers were driven by the quest to understand why certain populations lived longer, healthier lives compared to others. This journey took them around the globe, learning from isolated communities that were defying the odds.

The concept of Blue Zones dates back to the early 2000s, when a team of researchers, led by demographer Michel Poulain and physician Gianni Pes, pinpointed a region in Sardinia, Italy, where an unusually high number of centenarians thrived. They noticed something extraordinary in these towns: people were reaching age 100 at remarkable rates, experiencing lower incidences of chronic diseases like heart disease and cancer. Poulain and Pes demarcated this region in blue ink on a map, coining the term "Blue Zone."

This discovery piqued the interest of Dan Buettner, a National Geographic Fellow and journalist, who saw immense potential in unraveling the secrets of these long-lived communities. Buettner expanded the research beyond Sardinia, investigating other regions that exhibited similar patterns of longevity. His work identified four additional Blue Zones: Okinawa in Japan, Nicoya Peninsula in Costa Rica, Ikaria in Greece, and Loma Linda in California, USA.

Each of these regions offered unique insights but shared common lifestyle practices. Buettner's comprehensive investigation took years of data collection, interviews, and meticulous analysis. Working alongside a dedicated team of scientists, gerontologists, and anthropologists, they identified nine key lifestyle habits, known as the Power 9. These habits include moving naturally, maintaining a plant-based diet, having a sense of purpose, managing stress, and being part of a supportive community.

One of the most compelling aspects of this research was its holistic approach. Instead of focusing solely on diet or exercise, it considered a wide range of factors that contributed to a longer, healthier life. This comprehensive methodology set Blue Zone research apart from other studies on longevity, providing a multi-dimensional understanding of what it takes to live well into old age.

Skepticism and challenges were part of the research journey. Critics questioned whether genetics played a more significant role than lifestyle. While it's true that genetics influence longevity, Blue Zones research emphasized that lifestyle choices could dramatically impact life expectancy and quality of life, even within genetically diverse populations. This perspective helped shift the public's focus from unavoidable genetic fate to actionable lifestyle choices.

The impact of Buettner's work extended far beyond academic and scientific circles. His findings were widely published in books, articles, and documentaries, inspiring millions of people to adopt healthier lifestyle habits. Communities across the world began to embrace the Blue Zones philosophy, implementing changes in their diets, social structures, and daily routines.

In 2009, Buettner launched the Blue Zones Project, an initiative aimed at transforming American cities into healthier environments by applying the principles uncovered in the original Blue Zones. Collaborating with local governments, schools, and businesses, the project made significant strides in improving public health. Towns that participated in the project reported reductions in healthcare costs, lowered obesity rates, and increased life expectancy.

Despite the progress, the journey of Blue Zones research continues. Scientists still explore the intricate web of factors that contribute to longevity. New technologies and methodologies offer deeper insights into the biological, environmental, and social elements that shape our lives. Ongoing studies aim to refine our understanding and application of the Blue Zones principles, ensuring they remain relevant in an ever-changing world.

Looking ahead, the potential of Blue Zones research to influence global health is immense. By advocating for sustainable, community-driven changes, it presents a model for tackling modern health crises. Whether it's through urban planning that encourages physical activity or policies that promote mental well-being, the principles stemming from Blue Zones studies provide a roadmap for healthier, happier communities.

In essence, the history of Blue Zones research is a testament to human curiosity and resilience. It underscores the power of scientific inquiry combined with a genuine desire to improve lives. By looking to these unique regions of the world, we've gained invaluable knowledge that continues to inspire healthier living on a global scale. The story of Blue Zones is far from over, and its legacy will undoubtedly shape the future of public health and well-being.

Why Blue Zones Matter

The concept of Blue Zones is not just a fascinating look at unique pockets of longevity around the world; it's a blueprint for living a life that's both long and well-lived. For anyone committed to improving their health and extending their lifespan, understanding why Blue Zones matter is essential. It's not simply about eating certain foods or adopting new habits; it's about comprehending and embracing a holistic approach to life.

One of the pivotal reasons Blue Zones are vital is their profound impact on our understanding of aging and health. Traditionally, many societies have equated aging with frailty and decline. Yet, the residents of Blue Zones challenge this notion head-on. By observing those who live healthy lives well into their 80s, 90s, and beyond, we gain insights into habits and mindsets that defy the conventional expectations of aging. This new perspective can liberate us from destructive stereotypes and empower us to live our later years with vitality and purpose.

Moreover, Blue Zones give us a tangible, evidence-based framework for longevity. In a world cluttered with often contradictory health advice, the practices observed in Blue Zones stand out due to their basis in rigorous research and real-life application. Dan Buettner and his team didn't just theorize these principles; they traveled, observed, and analyzed communities like Okinawa in Japan, Sardinia in Italy, and Loma Linda in California. They cataloged the commonalities that contribute to their remarkable health and longevity.

Additionally, Blue Zones matter because they underscore the importance of community and connection. In our rapidly modernizing and increasingly isolated world, we often overlook the power of social networks and supportive relationships. Blue Zone inhabitants benefit immensely from robust family ties, strong friendships, and active communities. These social structures offer emotional support, a sense of belonging, and shared responsibilities, all of which play critical roles in health and well-being. Simply put, connection is a form of medicine we can't afford to neglect.

It's also critical to note the demonstration of dietary habits in Blue Zones. While many diets come and go in popular culture, often laden with extreme restrictions or obscure recommendations, the diets in Blue Zones are simple, accessible, and proven. People in these areas consume primarily plant-based foods, opting for vegetables, legumes, whole grains, and occasionally fish or meat. Moderation prevails over excess, guiding us towards balanced, nutritious meals.

The inherent wisdom of Blue Zones lies in their integration of physical activity into the fabric of daily life. Residents don't necessarily hit the gym or follow structured workouts. Instead, they move naturally throughout the day. Whether it's through gardening, walking, or daily chores, such regular, low-intensity activities keep them agile and fit. This seamless incorporation of movement is a practical lesson for anyone aiming to incorporate more physical activity into their hectic lifestyle.

Driving home the importance of purpose, inhabitants of Blue Zones display an acute understanding of why they wake up each morning. Whether it's the Japanese concept of "ikigai" or the similar notion of "plan de vida" in Costa Rica's Nicoya Peninsula, having a clear sense of purpose adds up to seven years of extra life expectancy. This sense of direction not only propels them forward but also provides a deep-seated sense of satisfaction and joy.

Another compelling reason for the importance of Blue Zones is the focus on stress reduction. Chronic stress is an insidious killer, linked to numerous health problems, from heart disease to mental illness. Blue Zone residents excel in managing stress through daily relaxation techniques such as meditation, prayer, napping, or simply enjoying a leisurely meal with loved ones. These habitual practices offer a natural buffer against the strains of modern living.

Blue Zones also challenge us to reconsider our environment and how it shapes our behavior. From urban planning that encourages walking to home designs that promote tranquility, the surroundings in Blue Zones are deliberately aligned to support a longer, healthier life. This insight pushes us to think beyond individual choices to the larger systems and environments that can foster or hinder our health goals.

Integrating spiritual practices into daily routines is another hallmark of Blue Zones that signals their significance. These practices are diverse, ranging from organized religion to personal rituals, but they provide a sense of peace, community, and existential security that nurtures mental and emotional well-being. Spirituality, in its many forms, acts as a linchpin holding the other elements of longevity together.

Sleep is yet another vital component highlighted by Blue Zones. The residents don't just get sleep; they enjoy restorative, quality sleep, which is critical for physical repair and mental clarity. This aspect of Blue Zones teaches us about the importance of sleep hygiene and the benefits of a restful environment. By following their example, we can improve our sleep and, consequently, our overall health.

Finally, Blue Zones matter because they present a holistic vision of healthy living that goes beyond the individual to encompass community and environment, proving that small, sustainable changes can have a massive impact. They show us that making these changes doesn't require a complete overhaul of our lives; instead, it involves adopting simple but effective strategies that are both sustainable and interconnected. This comprehensive model is empowering, urging us to take actionable steps toward a healthier, more fulfilling life.

Each of these aspects underscores the practicality and necessity of the wisdom gleaned from Blue Zones. By adapting these timeless practices to our modern lives, we don't just aim to add years to our lives but add life to our years. The science is clear and the stories compelling, invoking us to take a holistic approach to health, longevity, and happiness.

Chapter 2:
The Power of Community

It's no secret that we thrive when we're connected to others. In the world's Blue Zones, where people live the longest and the healthiest lives, community often plays a critical role. A strong social network provides not only emotional support but also practical help and a sense of belonging. By consistently engaging with family, friends, and neighbors, individuals reinforce positive behaviors, share healthy meals, and keep each other motivated. This sense of interconnectedness cultivates a support system that promotes well-being and longevity more effectively than isolated efforts ever could. To truly enhance your life and longevity, nurturing these relationships is as essential as a balanced diet or regular exercise.

Social Structures

The strength and cohesion of a community directly impact its members' health and longevity. Social structures, from tight-knit families to supportive networks of friends, form the bedrock of communities where people thrive into old age. When we observe populations in Blue Zones, these regions where people live significantly longer than average, we see how deeply interwoven social bonds contribute to their vitality and health.

Consider the role of intergenerational homes seen in many Blue Zones. These are not just living arrangements born out of necessity; they are deliberate choices that strengthen family bonds. Grandparents live with their children and grandchildren, sharing wisdom and providing emotional and practical support. This setup ensures that the younger generation benefits from the experience and care of the older one, while elders gain a renewed sense of purpose and belonging. There's a mutual benefit that stems from these living scenarios, offering an antidote to the isolation that plagues so many societies today.

Communities in Blue Zones also exhibit a remarkable tendency to prioritize regular, meaningful gatherings. From daily meetups for a cup of coffee to weekly communal meals, these interactions transcend casual conversation. They serve as a social glue that fortifies emotional support systems. In places like Okinawa, Japan, for example, the concept of "moai" involves small groups of people who commit to supporting each other for life. This formalized yet intimate network acts as an extended family, providing crucial emotional and sometimes even financial support.

Equally compelling is the impact of communal work and shared responsibilities. In regions like Sardinia, Italy, you'll find that community members often engage in agricultural activities together. This isn't merely about efficiency in completing tasks but more profoundly about reinforcing social ties and shared purpose. Working together toward common goals encourages a sense of interdependence and mutual respect, both critical elements in the fabric of lasting social structures.

Strong communities also excel in creating a sense of belonging and acceptance, which is indispensable for mental health. People who feel they are part of a supportive network are less likely to experience loneliness and depression, conditions that can have severe ramifications on physical health. Regular social interactions provide emotional validation and reduce stress levels, which in turn lowers the risk of chronic diseases. The mere act of knowing someone cares can create a powerful buffer against life's inevitable challenges.

Contrast this with the often fragmented social structures found in more industrialized societies where individuals may feel isolated despite being surrounded by millions of people. The erosion of community ties, fueled by hyper-individualism and a fast-paced lifestyle, contributes to declining mental and physical health. Reinforcing social structures can counteract these trends. Reintegrating communal activities, fostering intergenerational interactions, and prioritizing face-to-face connectivity can significantly improve our collective and individual well-being.

Of course, fostering such social structures in a modern, often fragmented society can be challenging. The key lies in intentionality and effort. Start small by cultivating connections within your immediate circle. Reconnect with family, make time for friends, and participate in community events. Volunteering is another meaningful way to build social bonds while contributing to the greater good. Whether it's at a local shelter, school, or community garden, the act of working together for a common cause can be deeply fulfilling and bind you to a network of like-minded individuals.

Moreover, workplaces can play a pivotal role in reinforcing social structures. Progressive companies are recognizing the importance of creating a community-like atmosphere within the workplace. Team-building activities, employee wellness programs, and communal spaces for breaks can foster a stronger sense of connection among employees. When people feel valued and part of a supportive network at work, their overall health benefits, and the positive effects spill over into other aspects of their lives.

The digital age, while often blamed for social isolation, also holds untapped potential for fostering connections. Online communities around shared interests or goals can provide critical support and a sense of belonging. Virtual groups, while lacking the depth of face-to-face interactions, can still offer a platform for exchanging ideas, providing emotional support, and building friendships. The idea is not to replace in-person interactions but to supplement them, creating a broader support network.

Spiritual and religious communities also offer robust social structures that contribute to longevity. These communities often emphasize compassion, altruism, and mutual support, providing a strong social safety net. Regular participation in group events, whether weekly services or community service projects, reinforces social bonds and offers a dependable source of emotional and sometimes even practical support.

Ultimately, the power of social structures lies in their ability to make individuals feel seen, heard, and valued. Feeling part of a community provides a sense of security and emotional well-being that is incomparable to any material possession. It's these social fabrics that bind us together, empowering us to lead healthier, more fulfilling lives. Investing in relationships and building robust social networks isn't just beneficial but essential for anyone seeking greater longevity and quality of life. Every effort to strengthen these social structures contributes to a healthier, more resilient community and, by extension, a more enriched existence for all its members.

Importance of Family and Friends

In our pursuit of longevity and a fulfilling life, the importance of family and friends can't be overstated. When we look at the world's Blue Zones, areas known for their high concentration of centenarians and remarkably low rates of chronic diseases, one critical commonality stands out: their strong social connections. These connections aren't just decorative ornaments on the Christmas tree of life; they're the sturdy branches that hold everything up.

Imagine the power of sitting down with family for a meal made from traditional recipes that have been passed down through generations. There's something almost magical about these shared moments. For one, they encourage you to slow down, cooking and eating together can foster a sense of belonging and purpose. Research has shown that people who feel connected to their families and communities tend to live longer and healthier lives. The moments you share over a kitchen table or on a weekend outing build the social fabric that brings meaning to our lives.

Relationships can act as a buffer against life's stresses, which, over time, can have measurable effects on your health. When stress strikes, knowing that you have a supportive network you can turn to reduces your cortisol levels, helping to keep your immune system strong. Cortisol, if chronically elevated, can wreak havoc on the body, leading to issues like heart disease and diabetes. But in communities where social ties are strong, such stress-related issues are less common. This isn't just anecdotal; it's grounded in scientific evidence.

It's not just about family, though. Friends enrich our lives in ways that even family sometimes can't. They provide perspectives that challenge us and help us grow. They empathize with our struggles and celebrate our triumphs. The Blue Zones are filled with tightly-knit friendship circles that often span a lifetime. In places like Okinawa, Japan, these social groups, called "moais," start at a young age and offer a lifelong sense of community and support.

Let's take a closer look at the sociocultural structures in Blue Zones. In Sardinia, Italy, it's common for multiple generations to live under one roof. This multi-generational living arrangement creates a strong support system. Elders instill wisdom and traditions in the younger generations, who, in turn, provide care and companionship. It's a win-win scenario that fosters emotional and physical well-being for everyone involved.

Friends and family can also help to keep you accountable for your lifestyle choices. If your peers are engaging in healthy behaviors, you're more likely to join in. Conversely, if they engage in unhealthy habits, you might be tempted to follow suit. This is the power of social influence. It underscores why creating and maintaining positive relationships is crucial for a long, healthy life.

In the context of health-conscious individuals striving for longevity, it may seem counterintuitive to focus on something as intangible as relationships when there are diets to follow and exercises to do. However, consider this: emotional well-being is deeply intertwined with physical health. Loneliness and social isolation have been linked to various health issues, including depression, cardiovascular disease, and even premature death.

Sometimes, the best prescriptions aren't pills but people. Engaging with friends and family can stimulate the release of oxytocin, a hormone that promotes bonding and reduces stress. In this way, your social life acts as a natural medication that you should take daily.

Let's not forget the importance of humor and shared joy. Laughter truly is the best medicine, and it's often shared in the company of others. Whether it's a light-hearted joke during a family dinner or a fun outing with friends, these shared moments of joy can lower blood pressure, boost immunity, and even alleviate pain. Laughter and light-heartedness foster a sense of community and connection, paving the way for a more resilient, positive outlook on life.

You might be wondering, "How can I build these kinds of robust, supportive relationships?" The answer lies in intentionality. Make a conscious effort to connect deeply with people. Scheduling regular family gatherings, joining community groups, or even volunteering can be meaningful ways to foster these relationships. Intentionally investing time and energy in building and maintaining your social network can yield dividends in terms of health and happiness.

Communication is a cornerstone of these relationships. Open, honest conversations help to build trust and understanding. Whether it's resolving conflicts or sharing aspirations, effective communication strengthens the ties that bind us together. Even simple acts like a phone call to check in on an elderly relative or a quick text message to a friend can make a difference.

In modern society, it's easy to get caught up in the hustle and bustle, prioritizing work and productivity over relationships. However, the sacrifices we make in our social lives can come at a high cost to our overall well-being. The lesson from Blue Zones is that no matter how busy life gets, investing in relationships should always be a top priority. The return on this investment is immeasurable and profoundly impacts our quality of life.

As you think about your goals for longevity and well-being, remember that family and friends aren't just part of the journey; they're the foundation. The power of community lies in these genuine, heartfelt connections. They're the glue that holds everything together, enabling us not just to live longer, but to live better.

So, as you take steps to enhance your diet, increase your physical activity, and reduce your stress, don't overlook the fundamental importance of family and friends. They enrich our lives in countless ways, providing the emotional nutrients that are just as vital as the physical ones. Embrace the power of these relationships, and in doing so, you'll be investing in a healthier, happier future.

Building Your Own Support Network

One of the most profound aspects of Blue Zones lies in the power of community. While smoothies and exercise routines can significantly impact your health, they pale in comparison to the influence that relationships with others bring into your life. In these regions, people are interwoven into tight-knit social structures that provide a web of support, encouragement, and shared purpose. To emulate this in your own life, you'll need to build your own support network.

We often underestimate the role that community plays in our well-being. But think about it. Who do you call when you're feeling down or need advice? Who do you share your joyous moments with? A strong support network can be the bedrock that holds everything together, allowing you to thrive both emotionally and physically. Without this, the journey to a healthier, longer life becomes significantly more arduous and lonely.

Creating a support network isn't just about making friends; it's about fostering relationships that are meaningful and mutually beneficial. Start by identifying the people who are already a part of your life. It could be your family, neighbors, coworkers, or members of clubs and organizations you belong to. These are your potential allies in this journey. Make a conscious effort to reach out to them. Share your goals and let them know how they can help you.

In Blue Zones, the concept of a support network extends to almost every facet of daily life. People often engage in regular social events, whether it's sharing meals, celebrating local festivals, or even casual gatherings like coffee meetups. These gatherings foster a sense of belonging and trust that is crucial for overall wellness. Emulating this practice, consider organizing regular get-togethers with your friends and family. It needn't be anything grand—Sunday dinners or a monthly book club can be just as effective. What's important is the regularity and the deepening of relationships.

It's also vital to diversify your network. Each individual you connect with brings unique strengths and perspectives, enriching your life in different ways. Some might offer emotional support, while others could bring practical advice or inspiration. Make it a point to develop relationships with people from different backgrounds, ages, and professions. This diversity will add richness to your interactions and broaden your viewpoint.

Moreover, volunteering is a powerful way to expand your social network while contributing to something bigger than yourself. Helping out in community projects or getting involved in local charities not only allows you to meet new people but also imbues your life with a sense of purpose and fulfillment. These shared experiences can forge strong bonds and bring like-minded individuals into your circle.

However, building a support network requires not just outreach but also introspection. To form strong bonds, you have to be a good friend yourself. Take the time to listen, really listen, when others speak. Show empathy and understanding. Be there for others not just during their highs but also their lows. This reciprocity forms the foundation of any meaningful relationship.

Sometimes, cultivating deeper connections may require you to step out of your comfort zone. If you're more introverted, pushing yourself to attend social events or initiate coffee meetups might feel daunting. But the benefits far outweigh the initial discomfort. As you take these steps, you'll likely find that others are also seeking the same kind of supportive relationships and will respond positively to your efforts.

Technology, often seen as a barrier to meaningful relationships, can also be a powerful enabler if used wisely. Engage in online communities that align with your interests and goals. Virtual book clubs, webinars, and social media groups can serve as platforms to meet new people who share your vision for a healthier, longer life. Just be mindful to balance online interactions with face-to-face meetings to keep the connections authentic and meaningful.

Also, don't underestimate the power of small gestures in strengthening your relationships. A simple "thank you" note, a birthday greeting, or checking in with someone who's having a rough day can make a huge difference. These seemingly minor acts accumulate over time, weaving a network of goodwill and trust that is indispensable.

It's equally important to establish some boundaries. While it's essential to be available and supportive, overextending yourself can lead to burnout, making you less effective in your interactions. Balancing your commitments ensures that you can sustain these relationships over the long term without compromising your own well-being.

Stress management also plays a crucial role in maintaining a healthy support network. High-stress levels can strain even the strongest relationships. Open communication about your stressors and actively seeking advice or assistance from your network can provide relief. Moreover, when your friends and family know what you're going through, they are more likely to offer the kind of support you need.

Ultimately, building a support network is not a one-time effort but a continuous process. As you grow and change, so too will your social needs and relationships. Periodically reassess your network to ensure it remains strong and supportive. Weed out toxic relationships and nurture those that bring positivity and growth into your life.

To sum up, creating a durable support network requires both effort and intention. But the rewards—improved mental health, increased longevity, and a profound sense of belonging—make it immensely worthwhile. So take that first step. Reach out, connect, and begin building the community that will walk with you on your journey to a healthier, happier life.

Chapter 3:
Diet and Nutrition

In exploring the secrets to longevity, diet and nutrition emerge as pivotal elements. Embracing a largely plant-based diet, rich in vegetables, fruits, legumes, nuts, and whole grains, not only fuels our bodies but also fortifies our spirit. It's more than just what you eat—it's the joy and tradition tied to preparing and sharing meals. Picture the vibrant, seasonal produce that graces the tables of Blue Zones communities, lending color and vitality to every dish. Flourishing health starts with mindful moderation, appreciating the wisdom of stopping when you're 80% full—a practice that enhances both satiety and appreciation of food. As we delve deeper, you'll find that adopting these time-tested dietary habits isn't about restriction, but about creating a nourishing, vibrant lifestyle that promises enduring wellness and joy.

Plant-Based Eating

Adopting a plant-based diet is a transformative step towards enhancing both your longevity and quality of life. The emphasis on plant-based eating within the context of diet and nutrition is not just a passing trend; it's a cornerstone of some of the world's healthiest diets. The communities in Blue Zones—regions known for their high concentration of centenarians—demonstrate how a diet rich in fruits, vegetables, legumes, and whole grains can lead to a longer, healthier life.

One might wonder why plant-based diets are so effective. The answer lies in the rich tapestry of nutrients found in plants. Fruits and vegetables are abundant in vitamins, minerals, antioxidants, and fiber, all of which contribute to optimal health. These nutrients help reduce inflammation, a key factor in many chronic diseases, and improve overall bodily function. Plants are rich in phytochemicals, compounds that help fight off cellular damage and oxidative stress.

Consider the diversity of foods at your disposal: colorful berries bursting with antioxidants, leafy greens laden with vitamins, and legumes that offer plant-based proteins. Each food item serves a unique role, forming a symphony of health benefits. Beyond the obvious physical benefits, a plant-based diet also aligns with many ethical and environmental values, adding another layer of personal satisfaction and global responsibility.

Moreover, plant-based eating promotes gut health. Your gut microbiome, the community of microorganisms living in your digestive tract, thrives on plant fibers. A healthy gut microbiome supports digestion and the immune system, and it can even influence your mood and mental health. Adding a variety of plant-based foods ensures that you feed your gut the right kinds of fibers, which in turn support a robust and resilient gut microbiome.

Let's talk about scalability and practicality. One common misconception is that plant-based eating is expensive or difficult to sustain. In reality, it can be both affordable and simple. Staples like beans, lentils, rice, and seasonal vegetables are not just budget-friendly, but also versatile. You can prepare a myriad of dishes ranging from soups and stews to salads and smoothies. Local farmer's markets can be a treasure trove of fresh produce, often at lower costs than supermarkets.

Then there's the social aspect of food, which is an underrated but incredibly significant facet of longevity. Sharing plant-based meals with family and friends can foster a sense of community and togetherness. It's not just about the nutrients; it's about the connection and emotional nourishment that come with enjoying meals together. Blue

Zones research reveals that people who eat mainly plant-based diets often do so within tight-knit communities that share in the preparation and consumption of food.

Don't underestimate the power of grains and legumes. These foods are foundational in many traditional diets around the world and are particularly prevalent in Blue Zones. Whole grains like quinoa, brown rice, and oats provide essential fiber and keep you feeling full longer. Legumes such as beans, lentils, and chickpeas are excellent sources of plant-based protein, making them great alternatives to meat. They've been linked to lower risks of heart disease, diabetes, and certain cancers.

It's essential to think creatively about incorporating more plants into your diet. Gone are the days of the bland salad and steamed broccoli as your only options. Think roasted vegetables garnished with an array of herbs and spices, hearty bean soups, and fruit parfaits. Each meal is an opportunity to experiment with new flavors and recipes, making the journey as enjoyable as it is beneficial. Playing around with herbs, spices, and different cooking methods can turn even the simplest vegetables into dishes bursting with flavor.

The transition to a plant-based diet doesn't have to be abrupt or all-encompassing. It can start with something as simple as "Meatless Mondays" or gradually increasing the portion of vegetables on your plate while reducing the amount of meat and processed foods. Make small, incremental changes that align with your current lifestyle and dietary preferences. Over time, these small shifts can lead to a significant transformation in your overall diet.

Another point of focus should be on mindfulness. Pay attention to how your body reacts to plant-based foods. You may notice improved digestion, increased energy levels, and even better skin. These changes serve as positive feedback, motivating you to continue on this path. The goal isn't to aim for perfection but to make conscious, consistent choices that align with your health goals.

Now, what about the question of protein? It's a myth that you need to consume animal products to get sufficient protein. Plant-based sources like beans, lentils, chickpeas, quinoa, tofu, and tempeh are more than sufficient to meet your protein needs. Think of a bowl of quinoa and black beans, a hearty lentil stew, or a tofu stir-fry. These dishes are nutrient-dense and filled with the protein your body requires.

In addition to the direct health benefits, there's also a ripple effect on mental well-being. Eating more plants can improve cognitive function and lower the risk of psychological conditions like depression and anxiety. These mental health benefits provide another compelling reason to embrace a plant-based diet. You're not just nourishing your body; you're also contributing to a more balanced and resilient mind.

Don't forget hydration, though. Many plant-based foods have high water content, which naturally helps in keeping you hydrated. Cucumbers, watermelon, oranges, and strawberries are excellent examples. Adequate hydration is crucial for all bodily functions, including digestion and nutrient absorption. Incorporating water-rich fruits and vegetables can contribute to your daily fluid intake, making hydration almost effortless.

The journey of adopting a plant-based diet is both a personal and communal experience. It's an opportunity to align your eating habits with your health goals, ethical values, and environmental concerns. The foods you choose to fuel your body not only affect you but also have broader implications for the planet. By opting for plant-based choices, you're contributing to a more sustainable world.

In conclusion, transitioning to a plant-based diet is a powerful step toward enhancing your longevity and improving your quality of life. Whether you're inspired by the Blue Zones or simply seeking to make healthier choices, embracing a variety of fruits, vegetables, grains, and legumes will pay dividends in health and happiness. Start small, stay committed, and you'll likely find this lifestyle not only beneficial but also deeply rewarding. By nourishing your body with vibrant, nutritional foods, you're setting the stage for a longer, healthier, and more fulfilling life.

Traditional Blue Zone Recipes

When we delve into the heart of Blue Zone regions, one of the most compelling aspects is their culinary traditions. These aren't just meals; they are reflections of a way of life, deeply rooted in community, seasonality, and balance. Traditional Blue Zone recipes offer a window into the dietary habits that contribute to the enviable longevity of these populations. They are simple yet nourishing, focusing on whole, unprocessed foods that support both body and soul.

Take, for example, the minestrone of Sardinia—a humble soup made with an array of local vegetables, beans, and just a hint of pasta. This dish is a microcosm of the Blue Zone philosophy: nutrient-dense ingredients that provide a medley of vitamins, fiber, and protein. It's often enjoyed as a communal meal, underscoring the role of social interaction in overall health.

Ingredients:

- 1 cup dried kidney beans
- 1/4 cup olive oil
- 1 onion, chopped
- 2 carrots, diced
- 2 celery stalks, diced
- 3 garlic cloves, minced
- 1 zucchini, diced
- 2 potatoes, diced

- 2 tomatoes, chopped
- Salt and pepper to taste
- 4 cups vegetable broth
- 1/2 cup small pasta

Instructions:

1. Soak the kidney beans overnight, then drain and rinse them.

2. In a large pot, heat the olive oil over medium heat. Add the onion, carrots, and celery; cook until softened.

3. Stir in the garlic, zucchini, potatoes, and tomatoes. Season with salt and pepper.

4. Add the vegetable broth and kidney beans. Bring to a boil, then reduce heat and let simmer for about 1.5 hours.

5. In the last 15 minutes of cooking, add the small pasta. Serve warm.

The minestrone is more than just a recipe; it's a practice in mindful, conscientious eating. The very act of preparing and sharing this meal is imbued with a sense of purpose and connection.

Okinawa, another Blue Zone, brings us the comfort of sweet potato and miso soup. This dish encapsulates the Okinawan diet's reliance on plant-based foods and fermented products, both of which are celebrated for their health benefits. Sweet potatoes are a powerhouse of vitamins and antioxidants, while miso, with its rich umami flavor, provides beneficial probiotics that promote gut health.

Ingredients:

- 2 large sweet potatoes, peeled and cubed
- 4 cups dashi stock (or vegetable broth)

- 1 small onion, sliced
- 2 tablespoons miso paste
- 2 green onions, chopped
- 1/2 cup tofu, cubed
- Salt to taste

Instructions:

1. Boil sweet potatoes in the dashi stock until tender.
2. Add the onion, cooking until softened.
3. In a small bowl, dissolve the miso paste in a bit of the soup broth, then return it to the pot.
4. Add tofu cubes and simmer for another 5 minutes.
5. Top with chopped green onions before serving.

The simplicity of this Okinawan dish belies its depth of flavor and nutritional prowess. It's a beautiful example of how traditional recipes adhere to Blue Zone principles: few ingredients, gentle preparation, and an emphasis on whole, nourishing foods.

Traveling to Nicoya, Costa Rica, we encounter the richness of the traditional black bean soup. Beans are a staple in many Blue Zone diets, valued for their protein content, fiber, and ability to stabilize blood sugar levels. This soup is hearty and satisfying, often paired with a fresh corn tortilla or a side of avocado, enhancing its nutritional profile.

Ingredients:

- 2 cups dried black beans
- 1 tablespoon olive oil
- 1 onion, diced
- 2 garlic cloves, minced

- 1 bell pepper, chopped
- 1 carrot, diced
- 1 teaspoon cumin
- Salt and pepper to taste
- 6 cups water or vegetable broth

Instructions:

1. Soak the black beans overnight, then drain and rinse.

2. In a large pot, heat the olive oil over medium heat. Add the onion, garlic, bell pepper, and carrot, cooking until softened.

3. Stir in the beans, cumin, and seasoning.

4. Add the water or broth, bringing to a boil. Lower the heat and let simmer for 1.5 to 2 hours, until beans are tender.

This black bean soup is more than food; it's a testament to how simplicity can yield profound nourishment. The Nicoyan tradition of combining beans with locally available vegetables creates a dish that's as wholesome as it is practical.

In Ikaria, Greece, the longevity diet is punctuated with dishes like chickpea stew, which makes regular appearances on the dinner table. Chickpeas are a fantastic source of plant-based protein and essential minerals like iron and magnesium. This stew harmonizes these nutritious legumes with the vibrant flavors of Mediterranean herbs and spices.

Ingredients:

- 2 cups dried chickpeas
- 1/4 cup olive oil
- 1 onion, chopped

- 3 garlic cloves, minced

- 2 bay leaves

- 1 teaspoon dried oregano

- Salt and pepper to taste

- 6 cups water or vegetable broth

- 1/2 lemon, juiced

Instructions:

1. Soak the chickpeas overnight, then drain and rinse.

2. In a large pot, heat the olive oil over medium heat. Add the onion, cooking until soft.

3. Stir in

Moderation in Meals

The path to a long and healthy life often winds through our dining tables. You don't need a complex roadmap, just a shift in how we perceive our plates. Research from across the globe, especially from Blue Zones—those remarkable regions where people live significantly longer—underscores the power of eating in moderation. Yet, what precisely is meant by moderation, and why is it so impactful?

Moderation in meals isn't just about portion control. It's a holistic approach that encompasses the timing, types, and even the emotional landscape of eating. When you adopt a moderate approach, you're essentially embracing balance—eating just enough to fuel your body while savoring your food, not over-indulging in it. It's about achieving a harmony that supports longevity and overall well-being.

Imagine sitting around a table in Okinawa, Japan, one of the esteemed Blue Zones, where elders recite "Hara Hachi Bu" — a Confucian teaching that reminds them to eat until they are 80% full. This simple yet profound practice can help prevent overeating and reduce stress on the digestive system. The Okinawan way teaches us the subtle art of listening to our bodies and respecting its natural cues.

A key aspect of moderation involves pacing your meals. When you eat slowly, savoring each bite, you're more likely to recognize when you're satisfied. Your body needs time to signal fullness to your brain, which is often delayed. Rushing through meals not only robs you of the pleasure of eating but can also lead to overeating and subsequent regret.

But let's not forget the emotional and social elements of moderation. Eating with family or friends can enhance your meal experience and help you eat more mindfully. Sociable meals encourage conversation, laughter, and slower eating, all of which contribute to less consumption and a more joyful dining experience. The communal aspect of eating is deeply ingrained in Blue Zones culture and significantly contributes to the overall well-being of these communities.

In the Western diet, it's easy to fall into the trap of oversized portions and an overabundance of choices. The key to moderation is simplifying. Opting for smaller plates, for instance, can naturally reduce the amount of food you consume. Moreover, limiting variety, especially of high-calorie or processed foods, can also play a crucial role. Instead, favor whole foods—vegetables, fruits, whole grains, and lean proteins—these make it easier to practice moderation since these foods are often more filling and nutrient-dense.

Domination by processed, calorie-dense foods is one of the main culprits behind overeating and various health problems. However, when you embrace a diet rich in whole, unprocessed foods, your body gets the nutrients it craves, which can inherently regulate your appetite. These are core practices observed in Blue Zones, where whole, nutrient-rich foods are the norms, and processed foods are the exception rather than the rule.

Timing also plays a pivotal role in moderation. Many Blue Zone inhabitants practice intermittent fasting or have their smallest meal in the late afternoon or early evening. This aligns with our body's natural circadian rhythms and can significantly benefit digestion, sleep, and overall metabolic health. It's not just what you eat but when you eat that matters.

The idea of "feast days" or occasional indulgences also aligns with the concept of balance. By allowing yourself the flexibility to enjoy special occasions or cherished treats without guilt, you're more likely to stick to a balanced diet over the long term. This approach prevents the all-or-nothing mentality that often leads to yo-yo dieting and unhealthy relationships with food.

It's essential to acknowledge that the journey to moderation can be deeply personal and different for everyone. Factors like age, activity level, and even genetic predispositions can influence what moderation looks like for you. Therefore, it's useful to regularly reassess and adjust your eating habits to align with your current life stage and health needs.

In conclusion, moderation in meals is not a rigid set of rules but a philosophy that fosters balance, mindfulness, and joy in eating. Embracing this approach can lead to better health, longevity, and an enriching dining experience. By learning from the Blue Zones, where moderation is woven into the fabric of daily life, we too can cultivate habits that promote a lifetime of wellness. Take small steps, make gradual changes, and remember that the journey toward better health is a marathon, not a sprint.

Chapter 4:
Moving Naturally

Embracing the art of moving naturally is a cornerstone of longevity, forming an integral part of daily routines in Blue Zones worldwide. Rather than hitting the gym for intense workouts, centenarians seamlessly integrate physical activity into their lives through gardening, walking, and household chores. It's less about forcing exercise and more about letting movement flow naturally throughout the day. This approach not only strengthens muscles and improves cardiovascular health, but also nurtures mental well-being by reducing stress and fostering a deeper connection with nature and community. By adopting these simple yet profound practices, you can transform your everyday tasks into opportunities for enhancing your health and lengthening your lifespan.

Daily Physical Activity

When we think of physical activity, images of grueling gym workouts and intense sporting events often come to mind. But, within the context of Blue Zones, daily physical activity takes on a more organic and integrated form. In these longevity hotspots, movement isn't something reserved for an hour at the gym; it's a natural and enjoyable part of everyday life. This simple, daily integration of physical activity is a cornerstone practice that boasts incredible benefits for both body and mind.

In Blue Zones like Okinawa, Sardinia, and Ikaria, the inhabitants are not necessarily running marathons or lifting heavy weights. Instead, they engage in natural movements—gardening, walking, cooking, or even dancing—all seamlessly woven into their day-to-day routine. This concept is both empowering and attainable for anyone looking to improve their health and longevity.

One of the most compelling aspects of daily physical activity in Blue Zones is its accessibility. You don't need special equipment or gym memberships. You can start with something as simple as walking. Walking is an incredibly effective form of exercise and resonates across all Blue Zones. Whether it's a leisurely stroll through a park or walking to the market, it's a habit that serves as a foundation for a healthy lifestyle. To make walking a regular part of your day, consider adopting some of the following habits:

- Walk to nearby destinations instead of driving.
- Take short, frequent walks throughout the day.
- Organize social events that involve walking, like walking meetings or group strolls.

In addition to walking, gardening is another prevalent activity in Blue Zones. It might seem mundane, but gardening is a full-body workout that also brings mental clarity and joy. When you garden, you're bending, reaching, digging, and lifting—all while enjoying the fresh air and sunshine. It creates an excellent context for exercise that feels less like a chore and more like a rewarding hobby.

Consider adding some simple gardening tasks to your routine. Even if you live in an urban area, you can start a small herb garden or participate in a community garden. Aim to spend at least 30 minutes a day tending to your plants. Not only will you be moving naturally, but you'll also reap the benefits of fresh produce and a meditative break from the hustle and bustle of life.

Household chores also play a significant role in keeping Blue Zone inhabitants active. Sweeping, mopping, cooking, and even washing dishes may seem like obligatory tasks, but they contribute significantly to one's daily physical activity quota. These routine activities, often dismissed as simple chores, can add up to a comprehensive, low-intensity workout over time. The next time you're doing household chores, remember that you're also doing something beneficial for your health and longevity.

Beyond chores and gardening, enjoy activities that engage both your body and mind, such as dancing, swimming, or even playing with your children or pets. Many Blue Zones inhabitants participate in traditional dances, which often serve as social activities too. These moments of joy and movement aren't just good for the body—they nourish the soul and foster community engagement.

For those needing more structure, incorporating natural exercises into your daily routine can be incredibly beneficial. These are simple, equipment-free exercises that can be performed anywhere, anytime. Examples include:

- **Squats:** Use your body weight to perform squats. They're excellent for strengthening legs and improving balance.

- **Push-ups:** Whether full push-ups or knee push-ups, this exercise engages multiple muscle groups.

- **Stretching:** Incorporate simple stretches to maintain flexibility and alleviate muscle tension.

- **Balancing exercises:** Stand on one leg or walk heel-to-toe to improve your balance and coordination.

Implementing these exercises into your daily life doesn't require a set routine. Do squats while brushing your teeth, sneak in a few push-ups during commercial breaks, or practice balancing while waiting for your coffee to brew. The key is to remain conscious of integrating movement throughout your day.

Moreover, understanding the importance of micro-movements can have a profound impact on overall health. In Blue Zones, people rarely sit for prolonged periods. They frequently change positions, stand up, stretch, and remain active. This frequent, low-intensity movement is crucial for maintaining mobility and preventing ailments associated with a sedentary lifestyle. Consider adopting habits that reduce extended periods of inactivity:

- Set a timer to remind yourself to stand up and move around every 30 minutes.
- Opt for a standing desk or try standing meetings.
- Engage in light stretching or walk around during phone calls.

Remember, the goal isn't to perform high-intensity workouts but to integrate more movement into your daily life. This approach is more sustainable and reduces the risk of burnout or injury. Ultimately, the best exercise is the one you enjoy and can maintain over the long term.

Many people find that wearing a pedometer or using a fitness tracker can be motivating. These devices offer a tangible way to measure your daily activity and set achievable goals. Strive for a minimum of 10,000 steps a day, but remember that any increase in movement is beneficial.

The evidence linking regular, natural physical activity to improved health and longevity is compelling. Numerous studies highlight that consistent, moderate exercise can reduce your risk of chronic diseases like heart disease, diabetes, and certain cancers. It also plays a crucial role in maintaining cognitive function as you age.

What's more, natural movement contributes to emotional well-being. Physical activity stimulates the release of endorphins—

chemicals in the brain that act as natural painkillers and mood eleva-tors. Regular movement can reduce stress, anxiety, and symptoms of depression. It's a powerful tool for both mental and physical health.

It's also worth noting that family and community play a significant role in promoting daily physical activity. In Blue Zones, physical activi-ty is often a social endeavor. Whether it's walking with friends, garden-ing with neighbors, or participating in communal dances, these activi-ties strengthen social bonds while encouraging a more active lifestyle. Consider how you can invite your family and friends to join you in these endeavors, making movement a joyful and shared experience.

Incorporating daily physical activity into your life might seem daunting, but it doesn't have to be. Start small and gradually build more movement into your daily routine. Walk more, sit less, and enjoy activities that keep you moving naturally throughout the day. By em-bracing this approach, you're not just adding years to your life; you're adding life to your years, enhancing both your longevity and overall quality of life.

The essence of daily physical activity is its simplicity. It doesn't re-quire expensive equipment, extensive time commitment, or drastic lifestyle changes. It's about making a series of small, sustainable ad-justments to the way you live. So take that first step, however small it may be, and let the journey to a more

Incorporating Movement into Everyday Life

When we think about exercise, images of treadmills, gyms, and regi-mented workout schedules often come to mind. However, in Blue Zones—those regions of the world where people live the longest and healthiest lives—exercise isn't a separate, scheduled activity. Instead, movement is organically woven into the fabric of daily life, enhancing longevity without the need for elaborate routines or specialized equipment.

So, how can you incorporate more natural movement into your everyday life? The key lies in rethinking your daily habits and routines, and making small, sustainable changes that promote physical activity. Start by evaluating your typical day. Do you sit for long periods at work? Are you driving when you could be walking or biking? Simple questions like these can reveal opportunities to add more movement without drastically altering your lifestyle.

Consider your commute. If possible, walk or bike to work instead of driving. If the distance is too great, try parking farther away from your destination or getting off public transportation a stop early. These small changes might not seem like much, but they add up over time and can significantly boost your daily physical activity.

Another effective strategy is to incorporate movement into your household chores. Gardening, vacuuming, and even washing dishes are all activities that keep you moving. In Blue Zones, many people tend gardens, not just for the fresh produce but also for the physical activity and the mental peace it brings. The beauty of these tasks is that they serve dual purposes: you complete necessary chores while also engaging in physical activity.

At work, take breaks to stand, stretch, or walk around. Use lunch breaks as an opportunity to get some fresh air and move. Standing desks and ergonomic office setups can also encourage better posture and more frequent movement. Even taking a few minutes every hour to stand up and stretch can make a difference in your overall activity levels and how you feel at the end of the day.

Social activities are another great way to incorporate movement. Plan active outings with friends and family, such as hiking, biking, or even a simple walk in the park. These activities not only foster stronger social connections, which are crucial for longevity, but also ensure that you are moving naturally and enjoyably. When exercise is combined with social interactions, it feels less like a chore and more like a joyful part of life.

Don't forget about integrating movement into your leisure time. Instead of sitting down for hours to watch TV or scroll through your phone, consider activities that get you moving. Dancing, playing a sport, or even just taking your pet for a walk can be fun ways to increase your physical activity without feeling like you are exercising.

One of the barriers to moving more is often convenience. We are accustomed to taking the easiest route possible: elevators instead of stairs, ordering in instead of walking to pick up food, or using robotic devices to clean our homes. Being mindful of these choices and consciously opting for the more active route can slowly but surely change your habits. For instance, using stairs instead of the elevator, or choosing to walk short distances rather than drive, helps integrate movement naturally into daily life.

Also, consider how your living space can support more movement. Arrange your home in a way that encourages physical activity. Having a small garden, setting up a yoga mat in your living room, or even placing frequently used items in different rooms can create more opportunities for movement. The idea is to make your environment conducive to staying active without deliberate effort.

Embracing hobbies that require physical exertion can also be beneficial. Whether it's dancing, martial arts, woodworking, or even playing a musical instrument, hobbies that require you to move help maintain a natural level of activity. These activities also offer a sense of accomplishment and joy, contributing to both mental and physical well-being.

Moreover, try to incorporate some form of natural exercise into your daily routine. This might include stretches upon waking up, a gentle yoga session before bed, or a walk after meals. These activities don't require special equipment or a significant time investment but can make a big difference in how you feel and function throughout the day.

For those with children, transforming family time into active time can be invaluable. Playing games, riding bikes together, or even engaging in friendly sports can set a positive example for the younger generation while keeping everyone active. Children naturally have a lot of energy, and harnessing this can be a fun way to incorporate more movement into your life while bonding as a family.

Always remember, the goal is not perfection but progress. Celebrate small wins and incremental changes. Over time, these small adjustments accumulate, leading to better health and greater longevity. The Blue Zones' approach teaches us that moving naturally isn't about forcing ourselves into grueling workouts. It's about making movement an enjoyable, integral part of our lives.

Imagine your life six months from now, where regular, natural movement is part of your routine. You'll likely feel more energetic, less stressed, and more connected to your environment and the people around you. These positive changes are the stepping stones to a healthier, longer life.

Incorporating movement into everyday life isn't just about physical health; it's about creating a lifestyle that supports your overall well-being. By making small, mindful changes, you can embrace a more active lifestyle that feels less like a chore and more like a natural, enjoyable part of your daily routine. This holistic approach to movement can profoundly impact your longevity and quality of life, bringing you one step closer to the vibrancy observed in the world's Blue Zones.

Examples of Natural Exercises

When we think of exercise, it's easy to conjure up images of gym routines, running on treadmills, or lifting weights. Yet, in the world's Blue

Zones, the longest-lived and healthiest people don't adhere to structured exercise regimes. Instead, they engage in what researchers call "natural movement." This is less about hitting the gym and more about integrating physical activity seamlessly into daily life. Let's explore some examples of these natural exercises and how they contribute to longevity and improved quality of life.

A primary example is walking, a fundamental form of human movement that requires no equipment and can be done anywhere. Residents of Blue Zones walk for various reasons: to run errands, visit friends, or simply enjoy their surroundings. In places like Okinawa, Japan, and Sardinia, Italy, it's not uncommon for individuals well into their nineties to walk several miles each day. This regular, low-intensity activity helps maintain cardiovascular health, supports metabolism, and fosters mental well-being.

Gardening is another popular form of natural exercise. Many Blue Zone inhabitants spend many hours each week tending to their gardens. This activity involves a range of movements—bending, stretching, squatting, lifting—that keep muscles toned and joints flexible. Moreover, gardening under the sun provides the body with essential vitamin D, while the proximity to soil bacteria can even improve mood and immune function. It's not just physical; it's hugely beneficial for mental health too.

In places like Ikaria, Greece, and Nicoya Peninsula, Costa Rica, people often engage in manual labor that most of us would typically hire others to do. Chopping wood, carrying water, and building structures not only contribute to a sense of purpose but also provide a full-body workout. These tasks require agility, strength, and coordination, keeping the body strong and resilient.

Housework, often considered a chore, can be a surprisingly efficient way to stay active. Activities like sweeping, mopping, and dusting can raise the heart rate and engage various muscle groups. In Blue

Zones, these tasks are performed regularly, providing a form of functional fitness that contributes to overall health without the need for a gym.

Another cornerstone of natural movement in Blue Zones is the practice of "active rest." Unlike passive rest, which involves sitting or lying down, active rest consists of light, voluntary activities. This could mean playing with grandchildren, dancing, or doing light stretches. These activities keep the body moving and blood circulating without the intensity of a workout, contributing to everyday physical maintenance.

Communal activities also play a significant role. In many Blue Zones, social gatherings often involve some form of movement. Traditional dances, social games, and group walks are examples where community bonding and physical exercise intersect. These activities not only enhance physical health but also foster a sense of belonging and joy—both crucial aspects of well-being and longevity.

Consider the example of traditional Okinawan dance. These dances are often performed at social gatherings and festivals, providing a fun way to stay active. Similarly, the Sardinians engage in circle dances during festivals, which not only get their bodies moving but also reinforce social bonds. The repetitive, rhythmic movements enhance balance, coordination, and cardiovascular health.

Another example comes from the Adventists in Loma Linda, California, where community work and volunteering are integral. Activities like organizing community events, participating in charity runs, or assisting in local projects keep individuals physically active and socially engaged. This blend of social participation and physical effort contributes to both physical and psychological health, creating a holistic approach to well-being.

For those looking to incorporate more natural movement into their lives, it's helpful to think beyond conventional exercise. Look for opportunities to walk instead of drive, take the stairs instead of the elevator, and engage in activities that require physical effort. Try taking a lunch break to walk around your neighborhood, or consider a weekend hiking trip to reconnect with nature. Even small changes, like standing while talking on the phone or using a standing desk, can make a significant difference over time.

The goal isn't to add more to your already busy schedule but rather to shift how you approach daily activities. By integrating movement naturally into your day, you make it an effortless part of your lifestyle. Think of it as investing in your long-term health, one step at a time.

Natural exercises inherently align with the rhythms of daily life, making them more sustainable in the long run. They don't require special equipment, memberships, or even a lot of time. Yet, their cumulative effect is powerful. These activities not only enhance physical fitness but also bring joy, reduce stress, and strengthen social bonds. Indeed, they embody the spirit of a lifestyle dedicated to natural well-being.

The beauty of natural movement lies in its simplicity and accessibility. Everyone, regardless of age or fitness level, can incorporate these practices into their lives. Start by identifying activities you enjoy and make a conscious effort to include them in your routine. Whether it's gardening, walking, playing with your children, or dancing at social gatherings, every bit of movement counts.

In conclusion, the secret to longevity and a healthier life might not lie in high-intensity workouts or strict fitness regimes but in the simple, consistent movements that make up our daily lives. By looking to the residents of Blue Zones, we can learn how natural exercises can be seamlessly integrated into our routines, leading to a more active, fulfilling, and long life. Remember, the journey to better health is a marathon, not a sprint, and every step you take in the right direction adds up.

Chapter 5:
Purpose and Meaning

As we transition into exploring "Purpose and Meaning," consider this an invitation to delve into the core of what drives us. The notion of ikigai, a Japanese term often translated to "reason for being," plays a pivotal role in unlocking longevity. It's not just about living longer; it's about living well, driven by a clear sense of why you wake up each morning. Purpose goes beyond the surface to affect our heart, brain, and emotional resilience. Discovering and nurturing this profound sense of purpose isn't a luxury; it's a necessity. It shapes our interactions, fuels our passions, and, crucially, offers a roadmap to a more fulfilling and extended life. Purpose transforms routine into ritual, suffering into strength, and ordinary acts into meaningful contributions. So, let's embark on this journey to not merely exist, but to live with intention and grace, enriching both our years and the quality within them.

Finding Your Ikigai

In the journey toward a longer and more fulfilling life, discovering your ikigai—the Japanese concept of "reason for being"—can be extraordinarily powerful. It's a notion deeply rooted in the culture of Okinawa, one of the well-researched Blue Zones. People there live longer and healthier lives partly because they have strong ikigai to anchor them.

So, what exactly is ikigai? At its core, ikigai represents the intersection of four primary elements: what you love, what you are good at, what the world needs, and what you can be paid for. It's that sweet spot where passion, mission, vocation, and profession converge. It's what gets you out of bed in the morning and keeps you energized throughout the day. When you find your ikigai, every moment feels meaningful.

However, finding your ikigai is not an overnight endeavor; it requires introspection and exploration. Start by asking yourself some fundamental questions: What are the activities that make time fly by for you? What skills come naturally to you? What are the things that people frequently ask for your help with? Reflecting on these questions helps you identify areas that merit deeper exploration.

One way to start this process is by creating a Venn diagram with the four elements of ikigai. Draw four circles, and in each circle, jot down the corresponding answers to: What you love, what you are good at, what the world needs, and what you can be paid for. Look for overlaps and start to see where these circles intersect. This intersection is where you'll find your ikigai.

Don't rush this process. It takes time to delve deeply into these aspects of your life. Consider keeping a journal where you jot down moments when you feel truly alive, skills you enjoy honing, and feedback from others about your strengths. Over time, patterns will emerge, guiding you closer to your ikigai.

Sometimes, finding your ikigai means reconnecting with passions and dreams from your past. Many people set aside things they love in the hustle and bustle of life. These might be hobbies, artistic pursuits, or dreams that were shelved in favor of more 'practical' paths. Revisiting these can reignite forgotten passions and uncover hidden strengths.

In Okinawa, elders often have a strong sense of purpose. They tend to the gardens, pass down traditions, and engage in meaningful community activities. Interestingly, having a purpose doesn't have to be grandiose. Small, everyday contributions also add up to a fulfilling ikigai. It could be something as simple as volunteering at a local shelter, mentoring youths, or even nurturing your family. What matters is that it provides a sense of fulfillment and integrates you into a larger community.

Scientific research backs up the beneficial effects of having a purpose. Studies show that people with a clear sense of purpose live longer and enjoy better mental health. They're more resilient to stress, have lower rates of heart disease, and even better cognitive function as they age. That's because having a purpose gives you a reason to care for yourself, stay active, and remain engaged with the world around you.

Moreover, your ikigai is not static; it may evolve as you grow. What serves as your life's purpose at one stage might shift as your experiences and circumstances change. That's perfectly okay. Flexibility is key. Re-evaluate your ikigai periodically to ensure that it still aligns with your innermost desires and external realities.

For those struggling to pinpoint their ikigai, engaging in new activities can be illuminating. Take up a new hobby, learn a new skill, or volunteer for a cause you've never supported before. Novel experiences can offer fresh perspectives, revealing hidden facets of yourself that you might not have discovered otherwise.

A critical part of this journey is to practice mindfulness. Being present in the moment allows you to tune into your feelings and reactions, giving you valuable insights into what truly makes you happy and fulfilled. Try incorporating mindfulness practices like meditation or deep-breathing exercises into your routine to help you remain grounded and focused.

Your ikigai will bring you joy and foster a profound sense of well-being. Its discovery is a journey worth embarking upon, holding the potential to greatly enhance your quality of life. This sense of purpose forms a cornerstone of the Blue Zones, and by finding your ikigai, you're not just adding years to your life but also life to your years.

Throughout this book, you'll find many strategies and practices designed to help you live longer and healthier lives. From diet and exercise to stress reduction and building a supportive community, each chapter offers insights that can also help you uncover aspects of your ikigai. Embrace these lessons, and let them guide you towards a life filled with purpose and meaning.

The Role of Purpose in Longevity

In the pursuit of a long and fulfilling life, uncovering your purpose can be just as vital as diet and exercise. Numerous studies have shown that individuals with a clear sense of purpose not only enjoy a richer quality of life but also tend to live longer. This sense of purpose acts as a powerful motivator, steering us toward healthier lifestyle choices and bolstering our overall well-being.

In places like the Blue Zones, where people often live well into their 90s and beyond, purpose is deeply embedded in daily life. This isn't mere coincidence; it's an integral part of the culture. People in these regions often have a well-defined reason to get up in the morning, what the Japanese call *ikigai*. Whether it's caring for grandchildren, working on a beloved hobby, or contributing to the community, purpose fuels their longevity.

But why does having a purpose have such a profound impact on our health? One explanation lies in the mind-body connection. When we feel that our lives have meaning, our mental state shifts positively. This improved mindset leads to lower levels of stress, depression, and anxiety—common conditions linked to shorter lifespans. A positive outlook can even influence physiological processes, boosting immune function and lowering inflammation.

Furthermore, a sense of purpose encourages healthier lifestyle choices. When individuals have something they are passionate about, they are more likely to take care of themselves to continue pursuing that passion. This often translates into better nutrition, more regular physical activity, and more effective stress management—all factors known to impact longevity positively. Purpose-driven individuals also tend to avoid harmful behaviors and are more resilient in the face of life's inevitable challenges.

Consider the social aspect as well. Purpose often involves connections with others, be it family, friends, or the broader community. These social bonds are another key factor in longevity found consistently across Blue Zones. Engaging with a community provides emotional support, encourages physical activity, and gives a sense of belonging—all of which support a longer, healthier life.

For many, the idea of finding a purpose might seem daunting. It's important to remember that purpose doesn't have to be grandiose. It doesn't have to mean discovering a cure for a disease or writing a bestseller. Your purpose can be simple, like nurturing relationships, engaging in creative pursuits, or volunteering. What matters is that it resonates with you personally and gives you a reason to get out of bed each morning.

Interestingly, the benefits of having a purpose are not confined to age. Studies have shown that individuals who cultivate a sense of purpose early in life tend to accumulate the advantages over the years. However, it's never too late to find your purpose. Even in later years, discovering or rekindling a sense of purpose can still yield significant health benefits.

So, how can you find your purpose? Start by reflecting on what brings you joy and fulfillment. Pay attention to the activities that make you lose track of time or the things you would do even if you weren't getting paid for them. Ask yourself what you want to contribute to the world. Sometimes, reflecting on past experiences and pinpointing moments when you felt most alive can provide clues to your purpose.

Another effective approach is to set goals that align with your values. When you set and achieve these goals, you often feel a sense of accomplishment and fulfillment, reinforcing your sense of purpose. Sharing these goals with others can also amplify the effect, adding layers of social engagement and accountability.

Remember, too, that your purpose can evolve over time. What drives you in your twenties might change by the time you reach your fifties or seventies, and that's perfectly okay. Being adaptable and open to new experiences allows your sense of purpose to grow with you, continuously contributing to your longevity.

Additionally, being part of something larger than oneself often instills a deeper sense of purpose. This could be involvement in community projects, environmental conservation efforts, or advocating for social justice. Such engagements not only provide meaning but also connect you with like-minded individuals, further enhancing your social network and overall well-being.

Educational and professional pursuits can also yield a sense of purpose. Lifelong learning keeps the mind sharp and opens up new pathways for passion and interest. Whether it's picking up a new skill, going back to school, or simply indulging in a hobby, these activities can all contribute to your sense of purpose and longevity.

For some, spirituality and faith play a crucial role in defining their purpose. Engaging in spiritual practices and rituals often helps individuals find deeper meaning in life, offering a broader perspective that can be incredibly fulfilling. These practices can provide comfort in difficult times and anchor a person's sense of identity and purpose.

Lastly, don't underestimate the power of small, daily actions in contributing to your sense of purpose. Simple routines like gardening, cooking, or walking the dog can provide moments of joy and fulfillment. When integrated into your lifestyle, these small actions accumulate, contributing to an overall sense of purpose and well-being.

As you journey towards a longer, healthier life, embracing your sense of purpose can be one of the most rewarding steps you take. It's a journey that promises not just more years, but better years. By weaving purpose into the fabric of your daily life, you enrich your existence, establish meaningful connections, and foster a robust, health-supportive mindset.

Creating a Purposeful Life

In embracing a life filled with both purpose and meaning, we step onto a path that leads not only to longevity but to a richer, more fulfilling existence. Purpose isn't an abstract concept confined to the realms of philosophy; it's a tangible force with the power to shape our everyday lives. When we have a strong sense of purpose, it becomes a driving force that propels us forward, giving us the strength and endurance to overcome life's challenges.

Purpose can be found in many places: in our careers, our relationships, our hobbies, and even in simple, everyday tasks. It's about identifying what gets you out of bed in the morning, what makes your heart sing, and what leaves you with a sense of satisfaction at the end of the day. For many, this starts with finding their *ikigai*, a Japanese term that translates to "reason for being." It's the intersection of what you love, what you are good at, what the world needs, and what you can be paid for. Finding this sweet spot can be transformative, turning ordinary days into extraordinary ones.

One way to begin creating a purposeful life is by reflecting on your values and passions. What activities make you lose track of time? What topics could you talk about for hours? Engaging in these activities and conversations can be incredibly fulfilling. Start by making a list of these passions and consider ways they can be incorporated into your daily routine. This doesn't necessarily mean a complete overhaul of your life; small, consistent changes can make a significant impact over time.

Another crucial component of a purposeful life is setting goals that align with your values. Goals give you something to strive for and provide a sense of direction. When your goals are aligned with your purpose, the effort needed to achieve them feels meaningful rather than burdensome. Break down larger goals into smaller, manageable tasks. Celebrate your progress along the way, recognizing that every step forward, no matter how small, is a step toward a more purposeful life.

Purpose and community are deeply intertwined. Surrounding yourself with people who share your values and passions can offer tremendous support and inspiration. Your community can help you stay focused on what matters most, providing encouragement during tough times and celebrating your successes. Seek out groups and communities where your purpose can thrive. This could be a local club, a volunteer organization, or an online community. The key is to find places where you feel a sense of belonging and where your purpose can flourish.

Furthermore, purpose can act as a buffer against the stressors of life. When you are engaged in meaningful work and activities, you're likely to experience lower levels of stress and anxiety. Purpose fosters resilience, giving you the capacity to bounce back from setbacks and maintain a positive outlook. It's not about eliminating problems but about having the strength to face them head-on.

Living with purpose also involves being present in the moment. Mindfulness and purpose go hand in hand; being fully engaged in whatever you're doing, whether it's a work project, a hobby, or a conversation, amplifies the sense of purpose. Practice mindfulness by paying attention to the present without judgment. This can be as simple as focusing on your breath, savoring a meal, or truly listening during a conversation. Over time, this practice can help to deepen your sense of purpose.

It's also important to recognize that your sense of purpose might evolve over time. What drives you in your twenties may be different from what fuels you in your forties or sixties. Allow yourself the flexibility to grow and adapt. Keep revisiting your values and passions, and be willing to make adjustments as necessary. This ongoing process of self-discovery is a vital part of living a purposeful life.

Journaling can be a powerful tool in this journey. By regularly writing down your thoughts, goals, and reflections, you create a concrete record of your purpose and progress. This practice can offer clarity and insight, helping you to recognize patterns and stay connected to your purpose. Spend a few minutes each day writing about what gave you a sense of purpose and what you experienced. Over time, you'll begin to see a clearer picture of what truly matters in your life.

Purpose doesn't always come with a lightning bolt of realization. Often, it's a gradual unfolding, a quiet revelation that comes from living with intention and mindfulness. Embrace the journey of discovering your purpose. Engage wholeheartedly with life, remain open to new experiences, and trust that your purpose will reveal itself in time. As you continue to build a purposeful life, remember to be kind to yourself, acknowledging the progress you have made and forgiving any missteps along the way.

A purposeful life is also a life of service. When we connect our purpose to something greater than ourselves, we unlock an even deeper level of fulfillment. Consider how your talents and passions can benefit others. Volunteering, mentoring, or simply being there for a friend in need can create a sense of purpose that is incredibly rewarding. These acts of service not only enrich the lives of others but also enhance your own well-being, creating a positive feedback loop of purpose and satisfaction.

As you cultivate a purposeful life, remember that the journey itself is as meaningful as the destination. Embrace the process of self-discovery and growth. Keep exploring what brings you joy and fulfillment, and don't be afraid to seek out new experiences. Life is a dynamic, ever-changing adventure, and your sense of purpose will evolve with it.

Lastly, share your journey with others. Talk about what gives you a sense of purpose and ask others about their passions and goals. These conversations can be incredibly inspiring and can help to foster a community of purpose-driven individuals. When we share our stories and support each other in our quests for meaning, we create a ripple effect that can transform not only our own lives but also the lives of those around us.

In the end, creating a purposeful life is about more than just adding years to your life; it's about adding life to your years. By finding and nurturing your purpose, you can lead a life that is not only longer but also richer, more fulfilling, and deeply meaningful. The journey to purpose is a lifelong endeavor, one that holds the promise of endless discovery, growth, and joy. Embrace this journey, and watch as your life transforms in ways you never imagined possible.

Chapter 6:
Stress Reduction

Stress, they say, is a silent killer, draining vitality and stealing precious years from our lives. By mastering stress reduction, we open the door to a longer, richer life filled with peace and purpose. Daily relaxation techniques, whether through meditation, deep breathing, or taking time to connect with nature, are the cornerstone of sustained tranquility. Beyond these practices, recognizing the importance of downtime and giving ourselves permission to rest without guilt can reinvigorate our spirits and recharge our minds. It's also essential to devise personalized strategies for managing stress, like engaging in hobbies, physical activities, or even seeking support from loved ones. Harnessing these tools not only diminishes stress but also cultivates resilience, ensuring we embrace each day with a calm, focused mind and a joyous heart.

Daily Relaxation Techniques

Finding ways to unwind and relieve stress every day is a cornerstone of a healthier, longer life. We're bombarded by stressors from all directions—work deadlines, family responsibilities, financial pressures. Taking daily steps to relax isn't a luxury; it's a necessity for living well. And it's not just about putting your feet up; it's about actively engaging in practices that calm your mind and body.

One effective technique is deep breathing. Engaging in a few minutes of deep, mindful breathing can drastically reduce stress levels.

It's simple: sit comfortably, close your eyes, and take a deep breath in through your nose, allowing your diaphragm to expand. Hold it for a few seconds, then exhale slowly through your mouth. Repeat this process for five to ten minutes daily. You'll find that this small practice can make a big difference in how you handle stress throughout the day.

Another excellent method is progressive muscle relaxation. This technique involves tensing and then slowly releasing each muscle group in your body, starting from your toes and working up to your head. It helps to physically release the tension you might not even realize you're holding. Begin by guiding your focus to each part of your body, one at a time. Tighten a muscle group, hold for a few seconds, and then let go. Feel the stress melt away as you systematically go through your entire body.

Mindfulness meditation can also be an invaluable tool. This practice isn't about emptying your mind but rather about acknowledging your thoughts without judgment and then letting them pass. You can start with just a few minutes a day. Sit quietly, focus on your breath, and observe any thoughts that come into your mind. Don't hold on to them; just let them drift away as you bring your attention back to your breathing. Over time, you can build this into a more extended practice, reaping increased mental clarity and emotional calm.

Engaging in physical activities is another fantastic way to unwind. Whether it's yoga, a short walk in nature, going for a swim, or even light stretching at home, these activities can dramatically lower cortisol levels, the body's primary stress hormone. Regular physical activity helps to reduce anxiety and depression, improves mood, and promotes a sense of overall well-being. It's about finding what you enjoy and making it part of your daily routine.

Sometimes, the simplest activities can provide the most relaxation. Reading a book, listening to your favorite music, or indulging in a creative hobby can serve as effective stress-relievers. If you find yourself perpetually caught up in daily hustle and bustle, carving out time for these activities can provide much-needed mental breaks. Even just a few minutes of doing something you love can make a substantial difference.

Another highly impactful technique is practicing gratitude. At the end of each day, take a few minutes to reflect on what you are thankful for. Write these down in a journal. The act of focusing on positive aspects of your life can shift your mindset and help you manage stress better. It trains your brain to look for positives rather than dwell on negatives, creating a buffer against stress.

For those seeking a deeper connection, spending time in nature can be incredibly therapeutic. The Japanese practice of 'shinrin-yoku,' or forest bathing, involves immersing oneself in the natural environment, allowing the sights, sounds, and smells of the forest to refresh and calm the mind. This practice has been shown to lower stress hormones, improve mood, and even boost the immune system. Even a simple walk in a local park can provide these benefits.

Technology can also aid relaxation when used mindfully. Numerous apps and online resources offer guided meditation, breathing exercises, and even virtual nature walks. These tools can be particularly helpful if you're new to relaxation techniques or need structured guidance to start. However, it's essential to balance screen time with real-world activities to avoid the stress that often comes with digital overuse.

Aromatherapy is another accessible method. Essential oils such as lavender, chamomile, and eucalyptus have been shown to promote relaxation and reduce stress. A few drops in a diffuser can create a calming atmosphere at home or work. You can also use these oils in a bath or apply them to your skin (properly diluted, of course). The soothing scents can help create a peaceful state of mind, making it easier to unwind.

Lastly, don't underestimate the power of human connection. Spending quality time with loved ones can be a significant stress-reliever. Whether it's having a heartfelt conversation, sharing a meal, or simply laughing together, these interactions can release oxytocin, the body's natural 'feel-good' hormone. They provide emotional support that can help you navigate life's challenges more effectively.

Incorporating these daily relaxation techniques into your routine requires intention and practice. Start with one or two methods that resonate with you and gradually build from there. The goal isn't perfection but consistency. As you dedicate time each day to relaxing, you will likely notice a positive shift in your overall well-being.

By committing to daily relaxation, you're not just combating stress; you're setting the foundation for a healthier, more balanced life. Each technique discussed can help you manage stress more effectively, improve your emotional health, and enhance your overall quality of life. Remember, these practices are tools at your disposal—use them to empower yourself and create a life filled with more calm, peace, and longevity.

Importance of Downtime

Taking time to unwind isn't just a luxury; it's a critical ingredient for a longer, healthier life. In today's fast-paced world, we're often swept up in a whirlwind of activities that leave little room for rest. But downtime, or periods of intentional rest and relaxation, can have profound effects on both our mental and physical health. Whether you're engaging in a hobby, spending time in nature, or simply lounging on your couch with a good book, making time for these moments can be transformative.

The importance of downtime can't be overstated when it comes to stress reduction. When we take breaks, our bodies and minds have the chance to recuperate from the constant demands placed on them. This isn't just about avoiding burnout; it's about giving your system the opportunity to reset. During downtime, our brains actually perform essential housekeeping tasks: consolidating memories, solving subconscious problems, and even making creative leaps.

Assuming moments of rest means breaking the cycle of constant stimulation. Our daily lives, flooded with notifications, emails, and the pressure to always be on, require counterbalance. Engaging in downtime may feel unproductive, but it paradoxically increases productivity and effectiveness over the long run. When we're well-rested and stress-free, we can approach tasks with more energy, focus, and creativity. The renewed sense of clarity and calm that comes from taking time off works wonders for problem-solving and decision-making.

Downtime also plays a vital role in our emotional well-being. Chronic stress can wreak havoc on our moods, contributing to anxiety, depression, and other mental health issues. Allocating time to relax and recharge allows us to manage stress better, making it easier to maintain a positive outlook on life. In essence, downtime provides the emotional and psychological resilience needed to navigate life's ups and downs.

Furthermore, downtime isn't just about relaxing in isolation; it often involves connecting with loved ones, engaging in leisurely activities, or simply enjoying the present moment. These moments of connection and mindfulness can lead to more satisfying relationships and a greater sense of community. Interaction without the pressure of tasks or deadlines brings authenticity and deeper understanding.

Downtime can take many forms, and what works best will vary from person to person. Some might find solace in meditation or yoga, while others might prefer a walk in the park, crafting, cooking, or spending time with friends and family. The key is to find what truly relaxes and rejuvenates you and to prioritize it regularly.

One practical way to incorporate more downtime is by setting boundaries. This might mean scheduling work-free evenings or weekends, turning off your phone at certain times, or designating specific areas of your home as stress-free zones. Creating these boundaries helps to ensure that downtime is respected and becomes an integral part of your routine, rather than an afterthought.

It's also worth considering the concept of "active rest"—activities that are low-stress but still involve engagement and movement. Gardening, gentle exercise, or even cooking a meal can serve as forms of active rest that offer relaxation without requiring complete stillness. These activities can be particularly effective because they combine physical movement with mental relaxation.

For many people, learning to embrace downtime requires a shift in mindset. In cultures that highly value productivity and busyness, it can be challenging to see rest as anything but wasted time. However, reframing downtime as a necessary part of a healthy, balanced life can bring a new perspective. Viewing relaxation as an essential activity, rather than a guilty pleasure, encourages us to incorporate it more willingly into our lives.

Historical and cross-cultural studies also underscore the importance of downtime. Communities that prioritize rest and leisure often report lower levels of stress and higher levels of well-being. These examples provide a compelling argument for the benefits of incorporating more downtime into our daily lives. Think of traditional siesta cultures or the Scandinavian concept of "hygge"—these practices all emphasize the value of relaxation and its integration into daily routines.

Ultimately, the benefits of downtime extend beyond mere relaxation. By making rest a priority, we allow ourselves to lead more balanced, fulfilling lives. We equip ourselves to handle life's challenges with greater resilience and foster better relationships with those around us. Downtime isn't just about escaping from the world—it's about recharging in ways that make us more present and engaged when we return to it.

The habit of making time for oneself can also inspire those around us to do the same. By modeling balanced behavior, we set a standard that fosters a culture of well-being. This can be particularly impactful within families and communities, creating a ripple effect of healthier, more balanced living.

So, take that break. Reserve those quiet moments. Recognize that in giving yourself some downtime, you're investing in a happier, healthier, and longer life. As you navigate through the various practices and insights presented in this book, remember to honor your need for relaxation. It's not just about living longer; it's about living well.

Strategies for Managing Stress

Stress is an inescapable part of life, but how we manage it can make a significant difference in our overall health and longevity. Effective stress management strategies aren't just about reducing stress; it's about transforming our relationship with stress and learning to harness it positively. In the Blue Zones, where people regularly live past 100, managing stress is a fundamental part of their daily routines. So, what can we learn from them?

Firstly, understanding that stress isn't always negative is crucial. It's our body's natural response to challenges and demands, preparing us to act. However, chronic stress can lead to serious health issues, ranging from cardiovascular diseases to mental health disorders. Therefore, adopting strategies to manage both the acute and chronic forms of stress can significantly improve quality of life.

One effective method for managing stress is through daily relaxation techniques. These could include practices like meditation, deep-breathing exercises, or progressive muscle relaxation. Even spending just a few minutes a day focused on relaxation can lower cortisol levels, the hormone associated with stress. In the Blue Zones, people often engage in meditative activities, whether it's through prayer, quiet contemplation, or mindful gardening.

Mindfulness and meditation have garnered a lot of attention for their stress-reducing benefits. They teach us to stay present and engaged, reducing the worry that often accompanies stressful situations. Studies show that regular meditation can rewire the brain to handle stress more effectively, enhance emotional health, and even improve sleep quality. Beginners can start with guided meditations available through various apps, gradually increasing their practice as they become more comfortable.

Social connections play a pivotal role in stress management. In the Blue Zones, people maintain strong family bonds and close-knit communities that provide emotional support during stressful times. Loneliness and social isolation can exacerbate stress, making it essential to cultivate meaningful relationships. Sharing your concerns with friends or family members can provide both emotional relief and practical solutions to problems.

An often overlooked but highly effective strategy is engaging in hobbies and leisure activities. Whether it's painting, gardening, or playing a musical instrument, hobbies provide an escape from daily stressors and a sense of accomplishment and joy. In the Blue Zones, people often engage in community activities that bring them together and give them a break from the rigors of daily life.

Regular physical activity is another cornerstone of stress management. Exercise releases endorphins, natural chemicals in the brain that act as painkillers and mood elevators. You don't have to be a gym enthusiast to reap these benefits; even walking for 30 minutes a day can significantly reduce stress levels. In the Blue Zones, physical activity is organically built into daily life, whether it's through farming, walking, or even dancing.

Nutrition also plays a role in stress management. A balanced diet rich in fruits, vegetables, and whole grains can impact mood and energy levels. Foods high in antioxidants, omega-3 fatty acids, and vitamins like B and D are particularly beneficial for alleviating stress. People in the Blue Zones often follow plant-based diets rich in these nutrients, which not only enhance physical health but also improve emotional well-being.

An essential yet frequently ignored aspect of stress management is adequate sleep. Poor sleep quality can increase stress levels and reduce the ability to cope with daily challenges. Establishing a consistent sleep schedule, creating a calming bedtime routine, and ensuring a restful sleeping environment can improve sleep quality and, in turn, reduce stress. In Blue Zones, people recognize the importance of rest and often take midday naps, contributing to their long-term health and longevity.

Time management and prioritization can also alleviate stress. By organizing tasks and setting realistic goals, you can reduce the overwhelming feeling that often accompanies a long to-do list. Learn to say no to non-essential commitments and delegate tasks when possible. In the Blue Zones, the pace of life is slower, allowing people to focus on what truly matters, reducing the constant rush and pressure that many of us experience daily.

Laughter and a sense of humor are natural stress relievers. Sharing a laugh can lower cortisol levels and enhance mood. In Blue Zones, people often come together for social gatherings, where laughter and joy are abundant. Whether it's watching a comedy show, reading a funny book, or simply spending time with a jovial friend, finding opportunities to laugh can significantly reduce stress.

Practicing gratitude can also shift your focus from what's stressing you to what's going well in your life. Keeping a gratitude journal or spending a few minutes each day reflecting on positive experiences can foster a more optimistic outlook. This mindset shift can reduce feelings of anxiety and depression, promoting a sense of well-being. In Blue Zones, many individuals regularly express gratitude, whether through prayer, meditation, or sharing their blessings with loved ones.

Lastly, seeking professional help should never be stigmatized. Therapists, counselors, and support groups can provide valuable insights and coping mechanisms for managing stress. Whether it's cognitive-behavioral therapy or simply having an unbiased person to talk to, professional help can be a crucial component of your stress management strategy.

Integrating these strategies into your daily life can create a balanced approach to managing stress. By taking cues from the Blue Zones, where managing stress is seamlessly embedded into daily routines, you can build a more resilient mind and body, paving the way for a healthier, longer life. Remember, the goal isn't to eliminate stress entirely but to develop the skills to manage it effectively, enhancing both your longevity and quality of life.

Chapter 7:
Lifestyle and Environment

Your environment can be a silent partner in your journey toward a longer, healthier life. The space you create around you, the spaces where you spend most of your time, can either uplift your spirit or weigh you down. Think about small yet impactful changes like adding more natural light, incorporating plants, and decluttering to create a more harmonious atmosphere. Sustainable living isn't just good for the planet; it's good for you too. By making eco-friendly choices, you contribute to a healthier planet and foster your own well-being. Imagine transforming your home into a personal Blue Zone, where every element— from the layout and design to the air quality and lighting— supports and enhances your health and happiness. Living sustainably and thoughtfully can turn your everyday surroundings into a sanctuary that nurtures both your body and soul.

Designing Your Surroundings

Designing your surroundings plays a pivotal role in achieving a longer, healthier life. It's no secret that our environment significantly influences our daily habits, attitudes, and overall well-being. For health-conscious individuals aiming to boost longevity through strategic lifestyle changes, curating a supportive environment can act as a catalyst for positive transformations. From your home to your workspace, every setting can be tailored to promote not just physical health but also mental and emotional resilience.

Consider starting with your home, the sanctuary where you retreat from the world. This should be a space that enables rather than inhibits your health goals. Think about the simple act of decluttering, which can have profound psychological benefits. A tidy space tends to reduce stress and make it easier to maintain healthy habits. Clear surfaces and organized belongings don't just look good—they make a strong statement about the kind of life you want to lead.

Now, envision how your kitchen could either support or sabotage your health goals. Placing healthier options at eye level in your pantry or refrigerator makes it easier to choose nutritious foods. You could also consider open shelving for displaying colorful fruits and vegetables, making them both visually appealing and readily accessible. The more appealing and reachable these items are, the more likely you are to consume them, thus integrating better nutrition into your daily life naturally.

A *well-designed living space* also includes areas dedicated to relaxation and mindfulness. Imagine a cozy corner with a yoga mat, some cushions, and perhaps a small fountain to add a soothing auditory element. This can be your go-to spot for unwinding and practicing mindfulness techniques after a busy day. And don't forget about lighting— natural light has been shown to improve mood and energy levels, so keep your windows unobstructed and consider strategically placing mirrors to amplify the daylight.

Connection with nature cannot be overstated. Whether it's a small balcony garden or a few potted plants inside your home, greenery has a calming effect and even improves air quality. Studies show that spending time in nature reduces stress, lowers blood pressure, and improves overall mental health. So, if possible, create an outdoor space that allows for interaction with nature. If an outdoor garden isn't feasible, bring the outside in with houseplants.

What about your workplace? Many of us spend a large portion of our days at work, making it another critical environment to consider. Ergonomic furniture can make a big difference in how you feel physically. Simple changes like a chair that supports good posture or a desk set up to minimize strain can prevent chronic discomfort and promote better productivity. If you can, make your workspace visually appealing—a clutter-free desk with some personal touches can uplift your mood and make the time spent working more enjoyable.

It's also beneficial to incorporate movement into your physical environment. Arrange your furniture to encourage frequent movement. Perhaps you place your printer across the room so you have to get up and move periodically, or you create a small area for stretching exercises. The idea is to make moving a natural part of your daily routine rather than something you have to schedule separately.

Another aspect of designing your surroundings relates to how you handle technology. We live in an age where screens dominate much of our day, often leading to issues such as eye strain and disrupted sleep patterns. Consider setting up a tech-free zone, particularly in your bedroom. Create a sanctuary for rest, free from the distractions of smartphones, tablets, and televisions. You'll likely find that your sleep quality improves, which in turn impacts every other aspect of your health.

In many Blue Zones, communal living and shared spaces promote social interaction and community support. While adopting a communal lifestyle might not be feasible for everyone, creating spaces that encourage social interactions can help. This can be as simple as a comfortable seating arrangement that fosters conversation or a dedicated space for family meals. When your surroundings support meaningful interactions, your emotional health gets a significant boost—one that contributes to a longer, happier life.

Let's not forget about sustainable living. Aligning your environment with sustainable practices isn't just good for the planet—it's good for you, too. Sustainable choices often have direct health benefits. For example, reducing plastic use can minimize your exposure to harmful chemicals. Prioritizing energy efficiency in your home often means better insulation and air quality. These seemingly small changes can collectively have a big impact on your well-being.

Lastly, consider the broader community settings you frequent, such as parks, cafés, and gyms. Aim to spend time in places that energize and inspire you. Seek out environments that reflect the values and lifestyle changes you aspire to incorporate. Joining a local club or participating in community activities can provide much-needed support and make your journey toward a healthier life more enjoyable and sustainable.

In summary, thoughtfully designing your surroundings can set the stage for a healthier, longer, and more fulfilling life. By making deliberate choices about your home, workplace, and broader community spaces, you create an environment that continually nudges you towards better habits and greater well-being. It's not about radical changes or expensive overhauls; it's about making intentional adjustments that align with your health goals. As you shape your environment to reflect these priorities, you'll find it easier to stay on the path to longevity and enjoy the journey along the way.

Sustainable Living

As we embark on the journey of sustainable living, it's essential to understand that this isn't just a buzzword or a fleeting trend. Sustainable living is a conscientious approach that deepens our connection to the environment and fortifies our health and well-being. It's about making choices that support long-term vitality, not only for ourselves but also for the planet we call home.

Think of sustainable living as a multigenerational plan. While it's tempting to focus solely on immediate benefits, the true power of this lifestyle lies in its long-reaching impact. By adopting practices that reduce our environmental footprint, we also pave the way for future generations to thrive. This chapter focuses on practical and actionable insights to adopt a sustainable lifestyle.

One cornerstone of sustainable living is a commitment to reducing waste. This goes beyond simple recycling; it's about rethinking our consumption habits altogether. Start by taking a closer look at what you buy and use daily. Are there areas where you can cut back? Simple swaps like using reusable bags, water bottles, and containers can significantly reduce daily waste. In turn, these practices benefit your health by minimizing exposure to harmful chemicals often found in single-use plastics.

Moreover, consider the provenance of your food. Sourcing locally not only supports community farmers but also reduces the carbon footprint associated with transporting goods over long distances. Local produce is fresher, more nutritious, and often organically grown, providing substantial health benefits. Farmers' markets are excellent places to find such produce. The immediate gain is evident in the quality and taste of the food you consume, enriching both your diet and your culinary experience.

Embracing a plant-based diet is another significant step toward sustainable living. This doesn't mean you have to become vegan or vegetarian overnight. Rather, focus on incorporating more plant-based meals into your weekly routine. Plants require fewer resources to cultivate compared to animal products, thus conserving water and reducing greenhouse gas emissions. From a health perspective, plant-based diets are rich in essential nutrients, providing numerous benefits like improved digestion and a reduced risk of chronic diseases.

Transitioning your home to be more energy-efficient can play a pivotal role in sustainable living. This involves both small changes and more substantial investments. Start with easy fixes like using energy-efficient light bulbs, unplugging devices when not in use, and opting for eco-friendly appliances. These changes not only reduce energy consumption but also lower your utility bills, making it a win-win situation.

If you're prepared to take bigger steps, consider investing in renewable energy sources such as solar panels. This can be a significant up-front cost, but the long-term savings, coupled with government incentives, make it a worthy consideration. More importantly, renewable energy reduces reliance on fossil fuels and decreases greenhouse gas emissions, contributing to a cleaner, healthier environment for everyone.

Water conservation is another critical element of sustainable living. Simple practices like fixing leaks, installing low-flow fixtures, and using a rain barrel can dramatically cut down water usage. Reducing water waste not only conserves this precious resource but also lessens the strain on local water treatment facilities. This has the added benefit of maintaining the natural beauty and health of local ecosystems, which directly impacts our well-being.

Creating green spaces within your living environment can also foster a sustainable lifestyle. Indoor plants improve air quality and add a sense of tranquility to your home. If you have outdoor space, consider starting a small garden. Growing your own herbs, vegetables, and fruits not only provides fresh produce but also offers physical activity and a sense of accomplishment. Gardening has been associated with reduced stress levels, improved mood, and a stronger connection to nature.

Additionally, the concept of minimalism goes hand-in-hand with sustainable living. The idea is to curate a life that prioritizes quality over quantity. Decluttering your space not only creates a more pleasant living environment but also leads to mindful consumption. You'll start valuing contentment and well-being over acquiring more material goods. This shift in mindset can lead to significant improvements in mental health, as a clutter-free space often translates to a clutter-free mind.

Transportation choices also have a massive impact on sustainability. Whenever possible, opt for public transportation, carpooling, biking, or walking. Not only do these choices reduce fossil fuel emissions, but they also contribute to your physical fitness. Walking or biking to work or the grocery store adds natural movement to your daily routine, complementing the principles discussed in the chapter on moving naturally.

Sustainable living isn't just about individual actions; it's also about community involvement. Participating in community-driven environmental initiatives can amplify your efforts. Local clean-up events, community gardens, and carpool networks are fantastic ways to engage with others who share your commitment to sustainability. This sense of community can provide emotional support and motivation, enriching your journey towards a sustainable lifestyle.

Ultimately, sustainable living is deeply intertwined with our quality of life. By taking steps to reduce waste, conserve resources, and make conscious consumption choices, we foster healthier environments. This, in turn, supports our physical health and emotional well-being. We're not just preserving the planet for future generations; we're enhancing our own longevity and the quality of our lives here and now.

As you continue to explore the various aspects of sustainable living, remember that this is a journey, not a destination. Start with small, manageable changes and gradually build up to more significant actions. Each step, no matter how small, contributes to a larger impact. Engage in this process with a spirit of curiosity and willingness to adapt, and you'll find that sustainable living isn't a chore—it's a fulfilling and enriching way of life.

Finally, keep in mind that every sustainable choice adds up. Whether it's choosing to bike to work, buy locally sourced produce, or simply unplugging unused electronics, your actions make a difference. Embrace sustainable living not just as a means to an end, but as a rewarding and empowering lifestyle that enhances your health, happiness, and connection to the world around you.

Creating a Blue Zone at Home

In the pursuit of longevity and improved quality of life, it's essential to create an environment that supports these goals. A Blue Zone at home isn't about drastic changes or expensive renovations. It's about thoughtful, intentional adjustments that foster well-being, promote healthy habits, and provide a sanctuary for relaxation and social connection. In this section, we'll explore practical steps you can take to transform your living space into your personalized Blue Zone.

One of the foundational principles of Blue Zones is the idea of designing your environment to make healthy choices effortless. Start by taking a critical look at your home layout. Are there areas that encourage sedentary activities over more active ones? Simple shifts, like positioning comfortable seating near natural light sources and creating designated spaces for hobbies and light exercises, can significantly impact your daily activity levels. For example, placing a yoga mat in your living room or setting up a small gardening area can remind and motivate you to maintain physical activity.

Next, consider the elements that bring calm and reduce stress. Stress management is crucial for longevity, and your home should be a sanctuary from life's daily pressures. Incorporate elements of nature, like indoor plants, which not only purify the air but also contribute to a tranquil atmosphere. Creating a small reading nook with soft lighting and comfortable seating or a meditation corner with minimal distractions can provide you with spaces dedicated to relaxation and mindfulness.

Organizing your kitchen is another key aspect of creating a Blue Zone at home. A well-organized kitchen, heavily stocked with whole grains, legumes, fresh fruits, and vegetables, encourages healthier eating habits. Arrange your pantry and fridge so that the healthiest items are within easy reach. This could mean placing fruits and vegetables at eye level and keeping healthy snacks like nuts or pre-cut veggies available. Cooking tools that make preparing wholesome meals easier, such as slow cookers and quality chopping boards, should be readily accessible.

Eating together as a family or with friends extends beyond just consumption; it builds social bonds and promotes better dietary practices. Incorporate a dining area that encourages shared meals. A large table, comfortable seating, and a pleasing aesthetic can entice everyone to gather for meals, enriching social connections and making mealtime something to look forward to. Avoid distractions during meals, such as TV or phones, to foster genuine conversations.

Your bedroom is another critical area for longevity. Quality sleep is a pillar of good health, and your bedroom should be conducive to restorative rest. Keep your sleeping environment cool, quiet, and dark. Invest in high-quality bedding and pillows to ensure comfort. If possible, follow a consistent bedtime routine and ditch electronic devices at least an hour before sleep, creating an ambiance that signals to your body that it's time to wind down.

Don't forget the importance of de-cluttering. A cluttered space can contribute to feelings of stress and overwhelm. Take time to declutter regularly, removing items that no longer serve you. This practice not only leads to a tidier home but also helps clear mental space. Donate, recycle, or repurpose items you don't need. Organize the rest in a way that maintains order and functionality.

Sustainable living is another aspect closely aligned with Blue Zone principles. Energy-efficient appliances, low-water-use fixtures, and incorporating renewable energy sources like solar panels are more than eco-friendly choices. They're investments in a sustainable future that also foster a life of purpose and mindfulness about our impact on the planet. Consider small steps like composting, using reusable bags, and minimizing single-use plastics to gradually transition to a more sustainable lifestyle.

Your home's social aspects shouldn't be overlooked. Creating inviting spaces for visitors can strengthen social bonds, which are integral to longevity. Whether it's a garden seating area, a cozy living room, or a back patio, these spaces should encourage interaction and connection. Hosting regular gatherings, even small ones like coffee dates or book clubs, can weave a social fabric that supports everyone's well-being.

Finally, consider how to personalize your space. Joy and satisfaction often stem from a sense of identity and belonging. Surround yourself with items that hold personal meaning and tell your story— family photos, travel souvenirs, or pieces of art that resonate with you. Personal touches don't just beautify a space; they anchor you to your life's journey and remind you of what's important.

Creating a Blue Zone at home isn't about drastic overhauls. It's about transforming your living space into an environment that advocates for longevity. Think of it as setting a stage where every prop and backdrop serves to enhance your life's performance. From mindful organization and de-cluttering to fostering connections and sustainable practices, the aim is to craft a home that's a reflection of a blue zone lifestyle. Every small change is a step toward a healthier, longer, and more purposeful life.

Chapter 8:
Faith and Spirituality

Faith and spirituality are often the invisible threads weaving through the tapestry of longevity and well-being in Blue Zones. They offer a sense of belonging, purpose, and peace that can mitigate stress and foster a resilient mindset. Many of the healthiest, longest-living communities are deeply rooted in spiritual practices, whether attending regular religious services, meditating, or simply taking time for daily reflection. These practices not only provide inner tranquility but also build social networks and emotional safety nets. To enhance your own journey toward longevity, consider creating small, meaningful spiritual routines that resonate with you. From moments of gratitude to structured rituals, these practices can nurture your spirit, enriching your quality of life and reinforcing the profound connection between faith, community, and enduring health.

Role of Faith in Longevity

Faith and spirituality often come up as powerful elements when discussing the broader dimensions of a healthy and long life. Our journey has taken us through diet, exercise, and mental well-being, but what about the impact of something less tangible yet profoundly influential—faith? At first glance, it might seem elusive to quantify faith's effect on longevity. Yet, research and anecdotal evidence from the world's longest-living communities reveal its undeniable role.

People who practice spiritual beliefs often possess a strong sense of purpose and belonging, both of which are crucial for mental health and overall well-being. These individuals are typically more resilient in the face of stress, knowing they have something greater to anchor them. This resilience is not just mental but physical. The immune system of spiritually engaged individuals often reflects their inner peace and balance. Being less susceptible to chronic stress, they maintain lower levels of inflammation and better cardiovascular health.

One of the most poignant examples is the role of faith in the Blue Zones—regions where people consistently live longer, healthier lives. In Okinawa, Japan, the spiritual practice of ancestor veneration fosters a deep sense of gratitude and responsibility. This embedded practice drives social cohesion, reduces stress, and provides a framework of purpose for daily living. Similar trends can be observed in Sardinia, Italy, where a predominantly Catholic population attends regular church services. Here, faith acts as a vessel for social interaction and communal support, both of which are beneficial to longevity.

Faith extends beyond traditional religious practices. Many find solace and purpose in non-religious spirituality through meditation, mindfulness, or simply a connection with nature. For instance, the Adventists in Loma Linda, California, a Blue Zone community, attribute part of their longevity to their faith in a higher power, paired with their healthy lifestyles. Their Sabbath observance offers a full day each week to decompress, connect with family, and practice gratitude—essential components of their holistic health approach.

Faith, in its various forms, often brings about routines and rituals that promote a structured life. Regular attendance of religious services or spiritual gatherings provides a sense of routine, which can be incredibly stabilizing. This structure isn't just about discipline; it creates opportunities for reflection, gratitude, and community bonding. Reflecting on one's life purpose, connecting with a higher power, or even participating in rituals can diminish feelings of isolation, one of the silent killers in modern society.

Moreover, faith communities offer an intrinsic support network. In times of crisis, having a group of like-minded individuals to turn to can significantly alleviate the burden. Shared beliefs and values create an environment where emotional support and practical help are readily available. This consistent social interaction mitigates loneliness and fosters mental health, which directly correlates to a longer lifespan.

Many might wonder if there is a direct causative link between faith and longevity. While faith itself might not magically extend one's years, the holistic benefits it brings—purpose, social interaction, stress alleviation, and healthier lifestyles—certainly contribute to a longer, more fulfilling life. Numerous studies indicate that individuals engaged in faith-based communities generally exhibit lower rates of depression, anxiety, and substance abuse. They're more likely to engage in preventative healthcare measures and maintain a positive outlook on life.

For our health-conscious readers seeking to enhance longevity through evidence-based lifestyle changes, incorporating elements of spirituality and faith can be immensely beneficial. You don't necessarily have to join a religious group; starting with small, intentional practices can make a difference. Daily meditation, regular reflection, or participating in community service projects can imbue your life with a sense of greater purpose and connectedness.

It's also essential to recognize that faith and spirituality can be deeply personal. What works for one person might not work for another, and that's okay. Find what resonates with you, whether it's a conventional religious practice, a personal spiritual journey, or a simple commitment to mindfulness and gratitude. The goal isn't to adhere to a strict doctrine but to cultivate a mindset that enriches your life and fosters resilience.

Embracing faith and spirituality doesn't need to be a grand endeavor. Small, consistent steps can build a foundation for lasting benefits. Consider integrating practices like daily affirmations, keeping a gratitude journal, or engaging in community activities. These practices may seem minor, but their cumulative impact can be significant, enhancing your quality of life while potentially adding years to it.

As you explore this dimension of well-being, remember that faith and spirituality are multifaceted. They provide a sense of peace, foster interpersonal connections, and create a framework for understanding and navigating life's challenges. By tapping into these elements, you empower yourself to face each day with renewed vigor, purpose, and a more profound sense of connection to the world around you.

In conclusion, faith and spirituality offer invaluable contributions to longevity. While diet and exercise are critical, the intangible benefits of a strong spiritual or faith-based practice enrich our lives in unique and powerful ways. They offer resilience, community, and purpose, all foundational to living a longer, healthier life. As you continue your journey towards enhanced longevity, consider the role faith and spirituality can play and how you might incorporate these elements into your daily life.

Life's journey is multifaceted, and while scientific evidence provides one lens, the intangible aspects of faith and spirituality offer another. Embrace both, and move forward with a balanced, holistic approach to a fulfilling, long life.

Let's journey on with the openness to embrace all avenues that can lead us to a prolonged, healthy, and meaningful life.

Spiritual Practices from Blue Zones

When we delve into the spiritual practices of Blue Zones, we uncover a tapestry of traditions, habits, and rituals that have supported not just longevity, but a more meaningful and connected way of living. In these regions, spirituality is not a separate compartment; it's woven seamlessly into daily life, offering a profound sense of purpose and community. In this chapter, we'll examine how these spiritual practices contribute to the health and happiness of Blue Zone inhabitants and explore ways you can integrate similar rituals into your own life.

One of the most impactful spiritual practices observed in Blue Zones is regular participation in faith-based gatherings. Whether it's attending a church service in Sardinia or joining a moai (social support group) in Okinawa, being part of a religious or spiritual community offers immense benefits. These gatherings provide emotional support, a shared sense of purpose, and a structured way to incorporate reflective and meditative practices into one's life.

For instance, in Loma Linda, California—home to a large community of Seventh-day Adventists—worship and social activities are intertwined. Worship services not only foster a sense of connection to the divine but also encourage strong community bonds, which reinforce healthy lifestyle choices. Such gatherings provide mental and emotional solace, and research suggests they can significantly reduce stress levels—a key factor in longevity.

Prayer and meditation are universal practices in Blue Zones, though they manifest in varied forms. For example, residents of Ikaria, Greece, often practice "chance" moments of prayer throughout the day, allowing for organic pauses that promote mindfulness and gratitude. This spontaneous approach contrasts with the structured, scheduled prayer times you might find in other cultures. Both methods, however, offer numerous health benefits, from reduced blood pressure to enhanced psychological well-being.

In Okinawa, the concept of "ichi-go ichi-e" (one time, one meeting) reminds people to appreciate the present moment and the uniqueness of each encounter. This spiritual mindfulness promotes a deeper connection with others and with oneself. It's a simple yet powerful practice: being fully present can reduce anxiety, improve emotional regulation, and foster a higher quality of life.

In Costa Rica's Nicoya Peninsula, daily spiritual practices often blend seamlessly with other wellness habits. Many locals begin their day with quiet, reflective activities, such as journaling or meditative gardening. Taking time for silent reflection allows them to set positive intentions for the day, grounding themselves in a sense of purpose and connection to the natural world.

Furthermore, rituals around food often carry a spiritual dimension in Blue Zones. Meals are more than just sustenance—they're opportunities for connection and thankfulness. For example, a simple act of giving thanks before meals, observed both in Nicoya and among the Adventists in Loma Linda, adds a layer of meaning to everyday activities. This gratitude practice contributes to emotional resilience and overall happiness by encouraging people to focus on the positives in their lives.

Religious and spiritual teachings in Blue Zones also promote healthy behaviors and ethical living. Many spiritual traditions advocate for moderation in all things, which aligns well with other longevity practices such as balanced nutrition and regular physical activity. Whether it's through dietary guidelines found in religious texts or the moral imperative to care for one's body as a temple, these teachings encourage a lifestyle conducive to long-term health.

Incorporating these spiritual practices into your own life doesn't require a complete overhaul of your current lifestyle. Simple steps can make a significant impact. Consider setting aside time each day for reflection, whether through prayer, meditation, or simple mindfulness exercises. Join or form a community group centered around shared spiritual or wellness goals, creating a support network that will enhance both your mental and physical health.

If you already belong to a religious or spiritual tradition, delve deeper into its teachings on health and well-being. Many traditions offer valuable insights into balanced living and stress reduction. If you're not religious, adopt practices that resonate with you from various traditions, like gratitude journaling, mindful eating, or community service. The key is consistency and finding what genuinely enhances your sense of well-being.

Ultimately, the spiritual practices from Blue Zones remind us that a longer, healthier life is profoundly interconnected with a sense of purpose, community, and inner peace. Embracing these principles can help you not only live longer but also foster a richer, more fulfilling life.

Incorporating Spirituality into Daily Life

Tapping into our spiritual side isn't just about finding solace during tough times; it's a powerful guide in our journey towards a longer, healthier life. To integrate spirituality into your daily existence seamlessly, it's important to understand that this isn't a one-size-fits-all concept. Your approach should be as unique as you are, respecting your beliefs and personal experiences.

First, consider beginning your day with a moment of mindfulness. You don't need to engage in complex meditation practices right from the start. Simply sit quietly, focus on your breathing, and set an intention for the day. This practice grounds you and aligns your actions with your core values. It's a small yet profound way to start your day with clarity and purpose.

Another accessible way to incorporate spirituality is through gratitude. Keeping a gratitude journal, for instance, can be a simple, daily practice. Each evening, jot down three things you're thankful for. They can be as small as a delicious cup of coffee or as significant as the support of a loved one. Gratitude shifts your focus from what's lacking to what's abundant in your life, fostering a positive mindset.

Engaging in regular communal or solitary prayer can also be deeply fulfilling. This doesn't necessarily have to be tied to a particular religion; it can be a moment of quiet reflection, sending out positive thoughts for yourself and others. Researchers have found that prayer and similar types of reflective practices can significantly reduce stress and enhance your emotional well-being.

Incorporating spiritual texts into your reading routine is another excellent method. Sacred scriptures, philosophical works, or books on spirituality can offer profound insights and moments of reflection. You might dedicate a few minutes each day to read passages that resonate with you, and ponder upon their meanings in the context of your life. This can be as much a mental exercise as it is a spiritual one.

Nature often serves as a powerful conduit for spirituality. Spending time outdoors, whether it's in a lush forest, beside a serene lake, or under a vast open sky, connects you to something larger than yourself. Take regular walks in nature, practice outdoor meditation, or simply sit in stillness, observing the world around you. Nature has a way of putting things into perspective, reminding you of life's interconnectedness and beauty.

Building a ritual around something you already enjoy can deepen your sense of spirituality. If you love cooking, make meal preparation a meditative activity. Savor the colors, textures, and aromas of the ingredients, and take a moment to be thankful for the nourishment they provide. If you're into art, let your creation be an expression of your inner world, a bridge between your spirit and the tangible universe.

Spirituality thrives on community as well. Joining a spiritual group or community not only strengthens your beliefs but also provides a support network. Whether it's a church group, a meditation circle, or a book club focused on spiritual texts, sharing your journey with others can be incredibly enriching. This connection fosters a sense of belonging, reminds you that you're not alone, and allows shared wisdom to flourish.

Let's not overlook the power of rituals. Daily rituals, big or small, punctuate your day with moments of meaning. Light a candle and say a prayer every evening, or brew your morning tea with a mindful presence. These small acts, repeated with intention, can transform the mundane into the sacred, bringing a soothing rhythm to your life.

Volunteering and acts of service also weave spirituality into the fabric of your day. Helping others not only contributes positively to the community but also enhances your sense of purpose and fulfillment. It's a powerful way to align your actions with your values, making your days more meaningful and your spirit more enriched.

Remember, spirituality and faith are not about grand gestures but about finding the sacred in the simple. It's about creating pockets of peace amidst the hustle and bustle, carving out moments of reflection in your day-to-day activities. It's about living in a way that's in tune with your inner self and the universe.

Maintaining a strong spiritual connection has been associated with numerous health benefits, including lower blood pressure, better immune function, and improved psychological health. It's not just an abstract concept but a tangible part of a holistic approach to longevity and well-being. Spiritual practices can reduce stress, a significant factor in many chronic conditions, thereby contributing to a healthier, longer life.

For many, spirituality also translates to inner resilience. Life is unpredictable, filled with ups and downs. A strong spiritual foundation can provide the mental and emotional fortitude needed to navigate life's challenges. It offers a sanctuary during storms, a reminder that there's more to existence than immediate worries and struggles.

So, as you embark on your journey to a healthier life, don't neglect the spiritual aspect. It's not merely an add-on but a crucial element of holistic well-being. Embrace practices that resonate with you, be consistent, and open yourself to the profound impact of a spiritually enriched life. This will not only help you achieve longevity but will do so in a manner where every moment is deeply felt and meaningfully lived.

Ultimately, incorporating spirituality into daily life is about fostering a deeper connection with yourself and the world around you. It's about reflecting on your values, finding beauty in the ordinary, and cultivating a sense of peace. This integrative approach ensures that as you work to extend your lifespan, you're also enriching the quality of those additional years. So, embrace the journey and let your spirit lead the way.

Chapter 9:
Sleep and Rest

In our fast-paced world, sleep often gets sidelined, yet it's a cornerstone of longevity and vitality. Getting quality rest isn't just for replenishing our energy; it's crucial for cognitive function, emotional well-being, and overall health. Blue Zone communities show us that integrating gentle, natural sleep habits into our lives can yield profound benefits. Simple practices like maintaining consistent sleep schedules, creating calming pre-sleep routines, and designing serene, comfortable sleep environments can drastically improve sleep quality. Achieving true rest requires more than merely closing our eyes; it's about fostering a life that values and prioritizes sleep. Embrace these practices, and you'll find that rest becomes a rejuvenating, cherished part of your daily rhythm, paving the way for a healthier, longer life.

Importance of Quality Sleep

When we think about extending our lifespan and improving our quality of life, diet and exercise typically top the list. However, often overlooked is an equally vital component: quality sleep. Many people may sacrifice sleep to squeeze more into their busy lives, but this trade-off can have profound consequences on both the body and the mind. It's not just about the quantity of sleep we're getting but the quality that stands as a cornerstone of good health and longevity.

Scientific evidence shows that sleep is indispensable for overall well-being. During sleep, our bodies undergo crucial processes such as cellular repair, hormone regulation, and detoxification. One of the lesser-known facts is that sleep helps regenerate our immune system. Think of it as a nightly tune-up that keeps our natural defenses sharp and ready to fend off illnesses. Indeed, the quality of our sleep can determine how resilient we are to common colds or more serious health conditions.

Memory consolidation and cognitive function are also closely tied to the quality of sleep. While we're restfully slumbering, our brains process and store new information, sorting and filing away memories like an efficient librarian. Compromised sleep can lead to decreased concentration, impaired decision-making, and slower reaction times. It's not an exaggeration to say that a good night's sleep sharpens the mind and prepares it for the challenges of the day ahead.

Hormonal balance is another aspect where sleep quality plays an indispensable role. Levels of critical hormones like cortisol, leptin, and ghrelin are regulated when we get sufficient sleep. Imbalances in these hormones can lead to increased stress, appetite irregularities, and ultimately weight gain. A well-regulated hormonal system contributes not just to physical health but also to emotional stability and mental clarity.

The cardiovascular system also greatly benefits from quality sleep. Research has shown that individuals who consistently experience poor sleep are at a higher risk for heart disease, hypertension, and even stroke. During deep sleep, the body reduces its heart rate and blood pressure, giving the cardiovascular system a much-needed break. This nightly respite is crucial in maintaining heart health and preventing chronic illnesses.

Beyond the physiological aspects, quality sleep contributes substantially to emotional and mental health. Insufficient sleep can exacerbate feelings of anxiety and depression, making it harder to face daily challenges and enjoy life's moments. Conversely, adequate rest equips us with the emotional resilience we need to navigate life's ups and downs. In essence, good sleep serves as an emotional reset button.

So how much sleep do we actually need for optimal health? While individual needs can vary, the general consensus among sleep experts is that adults should aim for 7-9 hours per night. However, this is not just about hitting a number. It's about ensuring that the sleep we do get is restful and of high quality. Deep, uninterrupted sleep cycles enable the body to go through all the necessary stages of sleep, from light sleep to deep sleep and REM sleep, each having its own set of benefits.

Unfortunately, modern lifestyles and environments can interfere with sleep quality. Exposure to artificial light, particularly blue light from screens, can disrupt our natural circadian rhythms. Consuming caffeine or alcohol late in the day can also hinder the ability to fall and stay asleep. Creating a sleep-conducive environment is essential. Simple changes like reducing screen time before bed, maintaining a cool room temperature, and investing in a comfortable mattress and pillows can go a long way.

The practices adopted by people in Blue Zones offer valuable lessons in prioritizing and enhancing sleep quality. For example, they often engage in physical activities throughout the day, which naturally leads to more restful sleep at night. They also tend to follow a consistent sleep schedule, going to bed and waking up at the same times each day, further stabilizing their circadian rhythms. Importantly, they integrate relaxation techniques such as meditation or evening walks, creating a seamless transition to a restful night.

One key takeaway from examining Blue Zones is the role of community and social support in promoting good sleep. Regular social interactions and a strong sense of belonging can alleviate stress and provide emotional comfort, enhancing overall sleep quality. In societies where people feel interconnected and supported, the likelihood of stress-induced sleep disorders diminishes significantly.

Quality sleep shouldn't be viewed as negotiable. It is a fundamental pillar of health that impacts everything from immune function and cognitive abilities to emotional well-being and cardiovascular health. Prioritizing sleep is a powerful, yet often underappreciated, strategy for achieving a healthier, longer life. Recognizing its importance and making conscious efforts to improve sleep quality can lead to transformative benefits, paving the way for a more vibrant and resilient you.

To conclude, integrating quality sleep into our daily health regimen is not merely an option; it's a necessity. The idea is not just to live longer but to live better. Good sleep empowers us to do exactly that. Embrace it, cherish it, and let it serve as the foundation upon which you build the rest of your longevity practices.

Blue Zone Sleep Practices

When we delve into the sleep habits of the world's longest-lived people, found in the Blue Zones, we discover a tapestry of simple yet profoundly effective practices. These practices contribute not only to their longevity but also to their overall quality of life. Learning from these centenarians, we can integrate these approaches into our own routines, enhancing both our health and our lifespan.

In Blue Zones, quality sleep is prioritized as an essential pillar of well-being. It's not merely about getting enough hours of rest but about the quality and consistency of those hours. Nightly rituals in these communities often include consistent bedtimes, conducive environments, and a focus on relaxation. This natural rhythm helps to reset their biological clocks, promoting restorative sleep.

A key takeaway is the power of simplicity. Many Blue Zone residents follow a pattern dictated by the natural world—they wake with the sun and wind down as it sets. This adherence to natural light cycles helps regulate their circadian rhythms, optimizing sleep quality. For those of us bound by the artificial lights and hectic schedules of modern life, this serves as a gentle reminder: aligning more closely with natural sleep-wake patterns can be beneficial.

Daytime napping is another common practice observed in Blue Zones. While some may view naps as a luxury, they're actually a necessity for many centenarians. Known as "siestas" in parts of the Mediterranean, these short rests rejuvenate the body and mind, reducing stress and enhancing overall functioning. Just 20-30 minutes in the afternoon can lead to marked improvements in alertness and productivity.

The environment in which one sleeps also plays a crucial role. In Blue Zones, bedrooms are sanctuaries designed for rest. Often, these spaces are free from electronic devices and excessive noise. Keeping your sleep environment cool, dark, and quiet can tremendously improve sleep quality, echoing the simple but effective strategies found in places like Sardinia and Okinawa.

Nutrition, too, impacts sleep. People in Blue Zones tend to consume their lightest meal at dinner, avoiding heavy, rich foods that might disrupt their rest. Alcohol and caffeine are consumed in moderation, and not too close to bedtime. Herbal teas, often with natural sedatives like chamomile or valerian root, are popular choices to aid in winding down.

Another fascinating aspect of Blue Zone sleep practices is the communal regard for rest. Resting isn't seen as a reward but a necessity. This cultural attitude towards sleep fosters an environment where it is normalized and respected. There is no glorification of overwork or sleeplessness; instead, sleep is celebrated as a cornerstone of health.

Many Blue Zone individuals also incorporate relaxation routines into their evenings, setting the stage for restful sleep. Whether it's a leisurely evening stroll, light stretching, or a relaxing bath, these activities signal to the body that it's time to unwind. These rituals are an integral part of their daily rhythm, reducing the buildup of daily stress and preparing the mind for sleep.

Physical activity, addressed more deeply in other chapters, is inherently tied to sleep quality. In Blue Zones, naturally incorporating movement into daily life ensures balanced energy expenditure. This natural exhaustion promotes deeper, more restorative sleep, a concept supported by countless studies linking physical activity with improved sleep.

The practice of mindfulness and meditation further enhances sleep quality in these regions. Whether through prayer, meditation, or mindful breathing exercises, these practices reduce stress and anxiety, common sleep disruptors. Techniques like these can be easily adapted into modern routines, providing a simple yet powerful tool for better sleep.

Learning to embrace a slower pace of life—a hallmark of Blue Zones—also has sleep benefits. Rushing through days with endless multitasking and engagements can lead to burnout and poor sleep. By cultivating a lifestyle that allows for downtime and reflection, as seen in these longevity hotspots, we can create a supportive environment for good sleep.

Finally, it's essential to acknowledge the role of social connections in sleep. Having a strong support network and a sense of belonging can significantly reduce stress levels, thereby improving sleep quality. In tight-knit Blue Zone communities, social interactions and relationships are integral, creating a support system that contributes to mental and emotional well-being, and by extension, better sleep.

In conclusion, adopting Blue Zone sleep practices involves more than just changes to our nightly routine—it requires a holistic approach to how we live our lives. By integrating these natural, time-honored practices, we can not only enhance our longevity but also enrich our quality of life. So let's honor our need for rest, embrace simplicity, and pave the way for healthier, more fulfilling days ahead.

Creating a Restful Environment

Creating a restful environment is immensely important for those striving to enhance their longevity and overall quality of life. Your sleep environment can either empower you to wake up refreshed and ready to conquer the day, or it can leave you feeling persistently groggy and unwell. A well-crafted sleep space not only promotes better sleep quality but also supports mental, emotional, and physical health in the long run. To start, let's explore key elements that cultivate a serene and restful sanctuary.

Your bedroom should serve as a haven, a retreat where all worries melt away. One of the foundational aspects is **decluttering**. A cluttered room often leads to a cluttered mind. When your bedroom is filled with piles of clothes, random gadgets, and unfinished projects, it breeds stress and distraction. Instead, aim for simplicity. Keep only essential items around and maintain a clean, organized space. This sense of order promotes calmness and reduces anxiety, creating a perfect backdrop for restful sleep.

Color choices also play a crucial role in setting the right mood. Soft, muted colors like cool blues, gentle greens, and subtle grays are particularly soothing. These colors can induce a sense of tranquility and peace, helping your mind to unwind naturally. It's best to avoid overly bright or highly saturated colors like reds and oranges, which can be stimulating and hinder your ability to relax.

Equally important is the **air quality** in your bedroom. Fresh, clean air can make a significant difference in how well you sleep. Consider investing in an air purifier to reduce allergens, dust, and pollutants. Additionally, integrating houseplants can not only beautify your space but also improve air quality. Plants like snake plants and peace lilies are especially effective in filtering indoor air and adding a touch of nature to your room.

Next, let's talk about *lighting*. Light significantly affects your circadian rhythm, which governs your sleep-wake cycle. During the day, exposure to natural light can enhance alertness and boost your mood. In the evening, however, it's crucial to dim the lights. Opt for soft, warm lighting and consider using blackout curtains to block any external light pollution from street lamps or early morning sun. This helps signal to your body that it's time to wind down and prepare for sleep.

The role of sound in your sleep environment shouldn't be overlooked either. While the world outside can be noisy and unpredictable, controlling the sounds within your bedroom is more feasible. White noise machines, calming music, or even nature sounds can mask disruptive noises and create a more tranquil atmosphere. Conversely, silence can be golden for some, making earplugs another viable option if you're a light sleeper.

Let's dive into the importance of your *bed*. Your bed is the centerpiece of your sleep environment, and its quality can make or break your sleep experience. A supportive mattress and comfortable pillows are non-negotiable for restful sleep. If you wake up with aches and pains, it may be time to reassess your bedding. Everyone's comfort needs are different, so whether you prefer a firm or soft mattress, ensure it aligns with your body's requirements.

Bedding materials also matter. Natural, breathable fabrics like cotton, linen, and bamboo can keep you cool and comfortable throughout the night. These materials are less likely to cause overheating, helping to maintain a stable body temperature, which is vital for uninterrupted slumber.

Temperature regulation in the bedroom is another key factor. According to sleep experts, the optimal sleep temperature is around 60-67 degrees Fahrenheit. A cooler room encourages your body to engage its own thermal regulation processes, promoting deeper sleep. During warmer months, ceiling fans, cool bedding materials, or even air conditioning can help. Meanwhile, during colder seasons, a warm but breathable blanket can make a world of difference.

Scents can also be powerful tools in creating a restful environment. Aromatherapy has been shown to improve sleep quality and duration. Essential oils like lavender, chamomile, and cedarwood have calming properties that can ease you into relaxation. A few drops on your pillow, or in a diffuser, can infuse your space with a gentle, soothing aroma.

Your nightly *routine* also plays a monumental role in fostering a restful environment. Consistency is key. Going to bed and waking up at the same time each day helps regulate your internal clock, making it easier to fall asleep and wake up naturally. Engaging in calming activities before bed, such as reading a book, gentle stretching, or practicing mindfulness exercises, can signal to your body that it's time to wind down.

Unplugging from electronic devices is just as important. The blue light emitted by phones, tablets, and computers can interfere with melatonin production, a hormone that regulates sleep. Make it a habit to switch off electronic devices at least an hour before bed. Instead, indulge in screen-free activities that relax your mind without overstimulating it.

Integrating these elements cohesively can transform your bedroom into a true restful haven. Establishing a sleep-friendly environment requires a bit of mindful planning and intentionality, but the rewards are well worth the effort. Enhanced sleep quality can boost your overall well-being, heighten your mood, and increase your longevity.

Remember, creating a restful environment encompasses more than just physical changes. It's about adopting a mindset that values rest as an essential component of health. By prioritizing a peaceful, conducive environment for sleep, you're laying the foundation for a more vibrant, healthful existence. It's an investment in your future self, one night at a time.

Chapter 10:
Healthy Habits

Building healthy habits is essential for enhancing both longevity and quality of life. As we've seen in our look at Blue Zones, the world's longest-living communities don't just passively achieve their good health; they actively cultivate it through small, consistent actions. These daily practices can range from mindful eating and regular movement to managing stress and fostering strong social connections. The key to establishing these habits lies in making them enjoyable and sustainable. By avoiding harmful behaviors and embracing positive routines, we can create a lifestyle that not only supports our health but also allows us to thrive. Start with one simple change and build from there; before you know it, you'll be well on your way to a healthier, more fulfilling life.

Positive Daily Practices

Establishing positive daily practices is a cornerstone of maintaining healthy habits and enhancing longevity. These practices aren't just about adding years to your life but also adding life to your years. They can seem minor at first glance but become incredibly impactful over time. Let's explore simple yet effective habits you can incorporate into your daily routine to build a healthier, more fulfilling life.

One of the simplest yet most powerful daily practices is starting your day with intention. Before diving into the hustle and bustle, take a few moments to set your goals for the day. This isn't just about creating a to-do list. It's about mentally preparing yourself for the day ahead, ensuring you approach each task with clarity and purpose. Doing so can significantly boost your productivity and reduce the likelihood of feeling overwhelmed.

Hydration is another fundamental practice that's often overlooked. Drinking an adequate amount of water daily is crucial for overall health. Water aids in digestion, maintains body temperature, and helps transport nutrients. Start your day with a glass of water and make sure to drink consistently throughout the day. Keep a water bottle with you to remind yourself to stay hydrated. This simple practice has long-term benefits, including improved skin health and better cognitive function.

Regular physical activity should also be a non-negotiable part of your daily routine. You don't need a gym membership or fancy equipment. Even a short walk can make a big difference. Movement, whether through walking, yoga, or even dancing around your living room, can boost your mood, improve cardiovascular health, and reduce the risk of chronic diseases. Aim for at least 30 minutes of physical activity daily to reap these benefits.

To ensure that these habits stick, it's helpful to incorporate them into a routine. Routines provide structure and predictability, making it easier to follow through on your positive daily practices. For instance, you might set a specific time each morning for a brief stretching session or a walk around your neighborhood. Creating these small daily rituals can make a big difference over time.

Mindfulness is another practice that can transform your daily life. Taking time to be fully present in the moment can reduce stress and anxiety, leading to better mental health. Whether through meditation, deep breathing exercises, or simply taking a moment to enjoy your surroundings, mindfulness practices can help you navigate the challenges of daily life with greater ease and calm.

Nutrition plays a crucial role in your daily practices as well. Opting for whole, unprocessed foods can provide you with the essential nutrients your body needs to function optimally. Start by making small changes, like including more fruits and vegetables in your meals. Over time, these small changes can add up and lead to a significant improvement in your overall health.

Social interactions are another key component of positive daily practices. Make it a point to connect with friends or family members each day, even if it's just a quick phone call or text message. These interactions provide emotional support and can significantly enhance your overall well-being. Remember, humans are social creatures, and nurturing these relationships is essential for a fulfilling life.

A gratitude practice is another powerful way to improve your mental health. Taking just a few moments each day to reflect on what you're grateful for can shift your focus from what's lacking in your life to what's abundant. This shift in perspective can improve your mood and overall outlook, making it easier to face daily challenges with a positive attitude.

Lastly, end your day with reflection. Take a few moments to look back on your day, acknowledging what went well and considering areas where you can improve. This practice not only helps you learn from your experiences but also sets you up for a better tomorrow.

Incorporating positive daily practices into your life doesn't require drastic changes. By making small, incremental adjustments, you can create a daily routine that promotes health, wellness, and longevity. The key is to remain consistent and committed, recognizing that these small steps, taken every day, can lead to significant long-term benefits.

Avoiding Harmful Behaviors

In our quest towards healthier living, recognizing and avoiding harmful behaviors is crucial. These behaviors, often habitual and subconscious, can undermine even the most robust efforts to adopt a healthier lifestyle. By identifying and actively distancing ourselves from these detrimental actions, we build a stronger foundation for lasting health and well-being.

First and foremost, let's address the omnipresent issue of smoking. Smokers significantly reduce their lifespan compared to non-smokers. The habit not only affects lung health but also increases the risk of heart disease, stroke, and various cancers. The sooner you quit, the better. If you've tried to quit before and didn't succeed, don't see it as a failure but as a learning experience. Each attempt gets you closer to your goal. Consider seeking support from healthcare professionals or smoking cessation programs - they can make a world of difference.

While most people are aware of the dangers of smoking, many underestimate the risks of excessive alcohol consumption. Moderation is key. A glass of wine with dinner can be part of a balanced lifestyle, but persistent overindulgence can lead to liver disease, mental health issues, and an increased risk of accidents. If you find it challenging to drink in moderation, it might be time to seek support. Sometimes, just talking to someone about your drinking habits can give a new perspective and provide the motivation needed to cut back.

Equally important is the avoidance of a sedentary lifestyle. Prolonged sitting has been linked to many adverse health outcomes, including obesity, Type 2 diabetes, cardiovascular disease, and even early death. Integrating more movement into your day doesn't mean you need to join a gym. Walking, gardening, dancing, or even taking the stairs more often can be incredibly beneficial. The goal is to keep moving naturally and consistently, as movement is integral to human health.

Mindless and emotional eating can also sabotage our health goals. Often, it's not just about what we eat, but why we eat. Stress, boredom, or emotions can drive us to consume unhealthy foods high in sugars, fats, and salt. Being mindful about food consumption, recognizing hunger cues, and finding healthy substitutes can curb this behavior. Mindful eating practices, such as eating slowly and savoring each bite, can reconnect us with our body's natural signals and promote healthier eating patterns.

Chronic sleep deprivation is another silent saboteur of good health. Consistently missing out on sleep can lead to serious health issues, such as impaired cognitive function, weight gain, and weakened immune function. Prioritizing sleep by creating a restful environment and establishing a regular sleep schedule helps to rebuild your body's natural rhythms and improve overall well-being. Remember, good sleep isn't a luxury; it's a necessity.

High-stress levels and poor stress management techniques deserve attention as well. Chronic stress can result in an array of health problems, including heart disease and weakened immune response. Implementing effective stress management strategies, such as meditation, deep breathing exercises, or even regular physical activity, can significantly lower stress levels. Don't hesitate to pursue activities that help you unwind and enjoy life; they're not just beneficial but essential.

Dietary choices extend beyond mindful eating to consuming food with integrity. Beware of highly processed foods loaded with artificial additives and preservatives. Instead, embrace a more natural diet rich in whole foods like fruits, vegetables, nuts, and grains. These not only provide the necessary nutrients your body needs but also reduce the intake of harmful substances that can contribute to long-term health problems.

Additionally, it's vital to moderate the intake of sugar and unhealthy fats. Excessive sugar consumption is linked to obesity, diabetes, and an increased risk of cardiovascular diseases. Unhealthy fats, particularly trans fats, can elevate bad cholesterol levels while lowering good cholesterol, increasing the risk of heart disease. Strive for a balanced diet that includes healthy fats found in avocados, nuts, and olive oil, and use natural sweeteners like honey or stevia when a sweet pinch is needed.

Technology, while a boon, can also be a bane if misused. The overuse of digital devices can lead to physical strain, sleep disturbances, and mental fatigue. Setting boundaries for screen time, engaging in digital detoxes, and ensuring that technology use doesn't infringe on your leisure and family time are critical. Establish tech-free zones or times, such as during meals or before bedtime, to foster healthier habits.

Social isolation can be easily overlooked but is a harmful behavior that can affect mental and emotional health. Building and maintaining strong social connections is essential for long-term well-being. Taking the time to nurture relationships, participating in community activities, and simply reaching out to friends or family can make a huge difference. Loneliness has been equated with smoking in terms of its impact on health, so don't underestimate the power of a connected life.

Lastly, toxic relationships and negative environments can severely impact mental and physical health. Surround yourself with positivity and supportive individuals who encourage and uplift you. Sometimes, the healthiest choice involves setting boundaries or stepping away from relationships that drain you rather than nourish you. Seek out environments and communities that foster mutual respect and growth.

To truly nurture longevity and a high quality of life, it's about making small, consistent changes. Recognizing the harmful behaviors that creep into our lives and actively working to replace them with positive habits boosts not only our lifespan but the joy we extract from each day. It's the combination of these mindful choices that carve the path to a healthier, more fulfilling life, one step at a time.

Establishing Healthy Routines

Establishing healthy routines is pivotal for anyone looking to lead a longer, more fulfilling life. While the idea of routines might seem mundane, they offer a powerful structure to support and sustain positive lifestyle changes. Think of routines as the backbone of well-being; they provide the consistency and predictability needed to maintain healthful habits over the long term.

One of the central elements of creating a beneficial routine is consistency. Consistency ensures that healthful behaviors become second nature. When something is done regularly, it transitions from being a task to becoming an intrinsic part of daily life. For instance, integrating a morning walk into your daily schedule can eventually become as automatic as brushing your teeth.

Start with small, manageable changes. It's tempting to overhaul everything at once, but sustainability comes from gradual shifts. Adding one new habit each week allows for adjustment without feeling overwhelmed. Consider beginning with something simple, like drinking more water or incorporating a five-minute meditation session into your morning routine. Over time, these small changes can compound to have a significant impact on your health.

Another key is personalization. What works for one person may not work for another, so it's essential to tailor routines to fit your unique lifestyle. Someone who enjoys mornings might schedule their exercise first thing, while a night owl might find post-dinner workouts more energizing. The goal is to create rituals that are enjoyable and can be maintained consistently, rather than forcing oneself into a template that doesn't quite fit.

Health-conscious individuals should also pay attention to balance when establishing routines. It's easy to focus solely on diet or exercise, but a well-rounded approach that includes mental health practices, relaxation, and social interactions is more holistic. For example, incorporating relaxation techniques, such as reading a book or practicing yoga, can play a significant role in reducing stress and improving overall well-being.

Accountability is another essential factor in establishing and adhering to healthy routines. Sharing your goals with a friend, family member, or even an online community can offer support and encouragement. Knowing that someone else is aware of your objectives creates a sense of responsibility, making it less likely that you'll skip your new habits when the initial motivation wanes.

The science behind behavioral change highlights the importance of triggers and rewards in forming new habits. A trigger is a cue that initiates the routine, while a reward reinforces the behavior. For example, placing a yoga mat next to your bed can serve as a trigger to practice yoga each morning. Following your session with a delicious, healthy breakfast acts as a reward, reinforcing the positive habit.

Setting specific goals and tracking progress can also help maintain healthy routines. Vague intentions like "get fit" or "eat better" can be discouraging due to their lack of clarity. Instead, aim for measurable and time-bound objectives, such as "walk 10,000 steps daily" or "include at least one serving of vegetables in every meal." Monitoring your progress, whether through a journal or a mobile app, provides tangible evidence of your achievements and can be motivating.

Another aspect to consider is flexibility. Life is unpredictable, and rigid routines can sometimes lead to stress rather than alleviate it. Allowing for some adaptability within your routines ensures that missing a day or two doesn't result in feelings of failure or demotivation. It's the accumulated effort over time that truly counts.

Establishing healthy routines is not just about self-discipline but also about enjoyment and fulfillment. Engaging in activities that bring joy boosts overall satisfaction and adherence to the routines. Whether it's cooking a new healthy recipe, taking a scenic route on your evening walk, or practicing hobbies that bring peace, find ways to derive pleasure from your daily habits.

Creating a supportive environment is crucial for maintaining healthy routines. Surrounding yourself with positive influences and minimizing exposure to negative ones can make a significant difference. This might mean reorganizing your kitchen to feature healthier foods prominently, or it could involve spending more time with people who share your health goals.

Morning and evening routines particularly benefit from careful planning. Your morning sets the tone for the rest of the day, so starting with activities that energize and focus you can improve productivity and mood. Similarly, an evening routine that includes winding down activities can enhance sleep quality, which is essential for overall health.

Incorporating mindfulness into your daily routines can also be incredibly beneficial. Mindfulness practices like meditation or simple breathing exercises can enhance mental clarity and emotional well-being. Even a few minutes of mindfulness each day can help reduce stress and improve focus, making it easier to adhere to other healthful practices.

It's easy to overlook the importance of self-compassion when establishing new routines. Being overly critical of oneself can lead to burnout and abandonment of healthful habits. Recognize that slip-ups are a normal part of the process, and instead of dwelling on them, focus on getting back on track.

Long-term success in establishing healthy routines often comes from viewing them as lifestyle changes rather than temporary measures. This mindset shifts the focus from short-term gains to enduring well-being, which is a more sustainable approach. Every small, consistent action contributes to a healthier, more fulfilling life.

There's a profound sense of empowerment that comes from being the architect of your health. Crafting routines that are meaningful and effective can transform daily life, infusing it with purpose and direction. These routines intertwine, reinforcing each other and creating a robust framework for longevity and vitality.

Ultimately, the journey of establishing healthy routines is deeply personal. It's about discovering what works best for you and making incremental changes that lead to lasting benefits. Embrace the process, stay flexible, and most importantly, enjoy the journey toward a healthier, longer life.

Chapter 11:
Scientific Insights

In the quest to extend not just the years in our lives but the life in our years, scientific insights offer invaluable guidance. Recent research on longevity reveals fascinating biological factors, including cellular mechanisms and genetic markers, that influence our lifespan and healthspan. Delving into this trove of knowledge, we find evidence supporting lifestyle choices that affect our genes' expression and metabolic health. The future holds promising directions in longevity science, from advancements in personalized medicine to innovative therapies targeting molecular pathways. This chapter integrates cutting-edge findings with practical advice, empowering you to harness science for a more vibrant, longer life.

Research on Longevity

The quest to extend human life has engaged scientists, researchers, and scholars for centuries. While the notion of immortality remains firmly in the realm of science fiction, significant advancements have been made in understanding the factors that contribute to a longer, healthier life. Modern research on longevity leverages a multidisciplinary approach, encompassing genetics, diet, physical activity, mental well-being, and socio-environmental factors.

At the forefront of longevity research are genetic studies. Twin studies, for example, have shown that genes can account for about 25% of the variance in human life span. This implies that while genetics play a crucial role, environmental factors are equally, if not more, significant. Researchers have identified specific genes associated with longevity, such as the FOXO3 gene, which has been linked to increased lifespan in diverse populations. However, inheriting such genes doesn't guarantee a longer life unless complemented by lifestyle choices and environmental factors.

Diet and nutrition remain pillars in longevity research as well. Mediterranean and Okinawan diets, both predominantly plant-based, have been associated with longer life spans and reduced incidence of chronic diseases. These diets are rich in antioxidants and anti-inflammatory compounds, which contribute to cellular health and reduced oxidative stress. Scientists continue to explore how specific nutrients and dietary patterns influence the aging process at the molecular level, including the role of caloric restriction and intermittent fasting in promoting longevity.

Physical activity is another critical area of focus. Regular, moderate exercise has been shown to extend life expectancy by reducing the risk of cardiovascular diseases, diabetes, and certain cancers. Research supports the notion that it's not about vigorous workouts alone; rather, daily, natural movements such as walking, gardening, or even household chores contribute significantly to longevity. Studies on communities with high concentrations of centenarians reveal that incorporating natural activity into daily routines is a common denominator.

Emerging evidence also highlights the importance of mental and emotional well-being in prolonging life. Chronic stress, anxiety, and depression can have detrimental effects on physical health, accelerating aging and increasing vulnerability to diseases. Longevity research underscores the importance of stress-reduction techniques such as mindfulness, meditation, and social connection. These practices help maintain cognitive function and emotional balance, critical components of a long, healthy life.

Sociological factors, such as social relationships and community, play an integral part in longevity research. Studies indicate that individuals with strong social networks and a sense of community live longer and healthier lives. Belonging to a supportive social group can provide emotional support, reduce stress, and encourage positive health behaviors. Research on Blue Zones, areas with high numbers of centenarians, consistently shows that social integration and communal activities are key longevity factors.

On the groundbreaking frontier of longevity science are advances in biotechnology and regenerative medicine. Stem cells, telomere extension, and even the prospect of gene editing with CRISPR are fields generating significant excitement. Researchers are delving into how they can harness these technologies to slow aging processes and repair or replace damaged tissues. While these are still in experimental stages, they offer a promising glimpse into the future of longevity science.

Additionally, the concept of "healthspan" versus lifespan is gaining traction in longevity research. Healthspan denotes the period of life spent in good health, free from chronic diseases and disabilities. Researchers are increasingly focusing on extending healthspan rather than merely increasing lifespan, ensuring that additional years of life are quality years. Interventions that improve healthspan, such as targeted therapies for chronic conditions and lifestyle modifications, are vital components of current longevity studies.

The role of sleep in longevity is another area receiving extensive attention. Poor sleep quality and sleep deprivation have been linked to numerous health issues, including obesity, heart disease, and reduced cognitive function. Ensuring adequate, restorative sleep is crucial for overall health. Researchers are investigating various aspects of sleep, such as duration, quality, and sleep disorders, to uncover their impacts on longevity.

Researchers are also looking into the potential of hormone therapies and supplements like NAD+ boosters, which show promise in reversing some signs of aging. While some of these interventions are still under investigation, they represent the cutting-edge possibilities in extending human health and life span.

Future directions in longevity research are incredibly exciting. Ongoing studies aim to understand better the complex interactions between our genes and environment. The burgeoning field of epigenetics, which studies how lifestyle and environmental factors can influence gene expression, is particularly promising. Epigenetic modifications hold the potential to turn on or off certain genes related to aging, which could be revolutionary in extending healthy life spans.

Despite these advances, it's essential to recognize that there's no one-size-fits-all approach to longevity. The interplay of genetic, environmental, and lifestyle factors is intricate and unique to each individual. Nevertheless, the findings from longevity research offer valuable insights and actionable strategies that can be adopted broadly to enhance the quality and duration of life.

In conclusion, research on longevity provides a robust framework for understanding how various factors contribute to a long, healthy life. From the genetic underpinnings to the critical role of diet, exercise, mental well-being, and social connections, the insights gained are invaluable. While the search for a Fountain of Youth might be an age-old quest, modern science brings us closer to meaningful, evidence-based practices that empower us to live longer, healthier lives.

Biological Factors

To understand the secrets of longevity and how we can harness them, it's crucial to dive deeply into the biological factors that influence our lifespan. Our bodies are extraordinary, complex systems influenced by a myriad of internal and external elements. These factors, studied extensively in scientific research, shed light on the potential for extending life and improving quality in our later years.

One of the most significant biological factors in longevity is genetics. While genetics certainly play a role, they aren't the whole story. Studies often cite that genetics may contribute to around 20-30% of aging's variance. Thus, although we inherit certain predispositions from our parents, our lifestyle choices play a monumental role in how these genes express themselves. This realization is empowering itself, suggesting that we possess considerable control over our own aging process.

Another critical component is cellular health. Human cells are equipped with telomeres—protective caps at the ends of chromosomes. Telomeres naturally shorten as cells divide, and when they become too short, cells can no longer divide and will either die or enter a state known as senescence. Various studies indicate that lifestyle choices affect telomere length. For instance, maintaining a healthy diet, exercising regularly, and managing stress can significantly slow down the shortening of these cellular caps.

What's equally fascinating is the role of autophagy, a process by which our cells clear out damaged components and recycle them into new cell parts. This cellular "housekeeping" is essential for maintaining cellular health and function. Techniques such as intermittent fasting have gained popularity due to their ability to trigger autophagy, thus contributing to cellular rejuvenation and extending lifespan.

Moreover, the balance of hormones in our bodies cannot be overstated. Hormones like insulin, human growth hormone (HGH), and cortisol each play intricate roles in regulating aging processes. Insulin sensitivity, for example, tends to decrease with age, leading to higher blood sugar levels and increased risk of type 2 diabetes. A balanced diet rich in whole foods, combined with regular physical activity, can help maintain insulin sensitivity, promoting a healthier aging process.

It's also important to discuss the impact of inflammation on aging. Chronic inflammation has been linked to a multitude of aging-related diseases, including heart disease, cancer, and Alzheimer's. Known as "inflammaging," this persistent, low-level inflammation accelerates the aging process. Anti-inflammatory diets rich in antioxidants, omega-3 fatty acids, and other anti-inflammatory compounds can mitigate these effects, underscoring the importance of dietary choices.

On a molecular level, there are certain proteins and enzymes that have been associated with longevity. One such protein is sirtuin, which influences cellular health and longevity. Sirtuins are believed to protect cells from dying and regulate the body's response to stress by affecting DNA repair mechanisms, cellular metabolism, and aging. Resveratrol, a compound found in red wine and certain berries, is known to activate sirtuin pathways, suggesting a potential pathway for dietary intervention in aging.

Exploring the realm of mitochondrial health reveals another cornerstone in the foundation of longevity. Mitochondria, the powerhouse of cells, are critical for energy production. As we age, mitochondrial function tends to decline, leading to reduced energy and increased vulnerability to metabolic disorders. Nutrient-dense diets, regular physical activity, and specific supplements like coenzyme Q10 can support mitochondrial function, fueling the body's cells more efficiently.

Let's not overlook the role of the microbiome either. The human gut houses trillions of bacteria that are instrumental in nearly every facet of health. An imbalanced microbiome is linked to a wide array of disorders, including obesity, diabetes, and even mental health issues. Probiotics, prebiotics, and a diet rich in fiber and fermented foods can promote a healthy microbiome, thus contributing to a longer, healthier life.

Interestingly, another area of longevity research is focusing on the role of epigenetics. This field explores how gene expression is influenced by environmental factors without changing the DNA sequence itself. Lifestyle choices such as diet, exercise, and even social interactions can trigger chemical changes that switch genes on or off, thereby influencing aging and longevity. Epigenetic mechanisms suggest that our everyday choices deeply impact gene expression, reinforcing the power of lifestyle in shaping our futures.

Senolytics, a newer area in longevity research, target senescent cells—cells that have stopped dividing and accumulate as we age, secreting harmful substances that induce inflammation and damage surrounding cells. Senolytic therapies aim to selectively clear these senescent cells, thereby improving health span and potentially increasing life span. Though still in their infancy, these therapies hold promise for future aging interventions.

Both calories and metabolism play nuanced roles in longevity. Caloric restriction has been shown in animal studies to extend lifespan significantly. While it's not entirely clear if humans will see the same benefit, moderate caloric restriction without malnutrition, often achieved through balanced nutrition and mindful eating, may offer health benefits. Additionally, metabolic health, including how efficiently our body converts food into energy, can influence the rate of aging. Maintaining an active lifestyle and a balanced diet helps to boost metabolic health.

Our understanding of biological factors is ever-evolving, continually providing new insights into how we can live longer, healthier lives. By embracing both the established and emerging science on these biological factors, we take steps not just to extend our years, but to fill them with health, vitality, and purpose. The journey to a longer life is not a distant dream but a tangible goal within our reach, grounded in our daily choices and habits.

Future Directions in Longevity Science

As we stand on the brink of unprecedented advancements, the future of longevity science presents an exhilarating frontier. Imagine a world where we don't just add years to life but life to years, making every moment more vibrant and meaningful. Emerging technologies and groundbreaking research promise to deepen our understanding and reshape the landscape of aging. For those committed to leading healthier, longer lives, staying abreast of these developments is not just intriguing but essential.

The integration of artificial intelligence (AI) and machine learning into medical research has already begun to change the way we understand aging. AI can analyze vast datasets far more quickly and accurately than traditional methods, uncovering patterns and insights that might otherwise go unnoticed. These technologies are being harnessed to identify biomarkers of aging, predict diseases before they manifest, and personalize treatments to an individual's unique genetic profile. As AI evolves, its role in longevity science will only expand, offering new tools to both researchers and healthcare providers in their quest to extend healthy lifespans.

Simultaneously, the field of genetics is making leaps and bounds. The mapping of the human genome has opened a treasure trove of information about the biological underpinnings of aging. Scientists are now able to identify specific genes that influence longevity and could potentially be targeted through gene therapy or other medical interventions. Companies are already working on therapies aimed at correcting DNA damage, enhancing cellular repair mechanisms, and even reversing age-related genetic changes. This line of research could eventually lead to treatments that slow down or even halt the aging process itself.

Equally exciting are advancements in regenerative medicine, particularly the use of stem cells. Stem cells have the unique ability to become any type of cell in the body, offering the potential to regenerate damaged tissues and organs. Clinical trials are currently underway to explore the viability of stem cell therapies for everything from heart disease to neurodegenerative conditions. If successful, these treatments could dramatically improve quality of life by repairing the damage that typically accumulates with age, allowing individuals to remain active and healthy for much longer periods.

The gut microbiome, the complex community of microorganisms living in our digestive tract, has also emerged as a key player in longevity. Recent studies have shown that the gut microbiome significantly influences immune function, inflammation, and even mood—all factors that impact aging. Researchers are exploring ways to modulate the microbiome through diet, probiotics, and even fecal transplants to promote a healthier, longer life. This area of research underscores the adage that we are indeed what we eat, and it has profound implications for how we might tailor our diets to foster longevity.

In the realm of pharmaceuticals, a new class of drugs known as senolytics is creating a buzz. Senolytics aim to clear senescent cells—cells that have stopped dividing but continue to secrete harmful substances, contributing to the aging process. Early studies in animals have shown that removing these cells can extend lifespan and improve healthspan, the time during which individuals are healthy and active. Human trials are currently in progress, and if successful, senolytics could become a powerful tool in our anti-aging arsenal.

On a broader scale, the concept of "aging in place" is gaining traction. With the integration of smart home technologies and telemedicine, it's becoming increasingly feasible for older adults to live independently while maintaining access to healthcare and social support. Innovations such as wearable health monitors, voice-activated assistants, and automated home systems are making it easier for seniors to manage their health and stay connected with their communities. These technologies not only enhance the quality of life but also offer valuable data that can be used to further longevity research.

The intersection of technology and biology isn't the only promising avenue. Lifestyle interventions, grounded in robust scientific evidence, remain fundamental to longevity. However, future directions could see these practices becoming even more refined and personalized. For instance, personalized nutrition plans based on one's genetic makeup and microbiome could become the norm. Likewise, exercise regimens tailored to an individual's health status and physical capabilities could optimize benefits. The goal is to move beyond one-size-fits-all recommendations to strategies that are as unique as the individuals who follow them.

Another exciting frontier is the exploration of the social determinants of health. Research has long indicated that factors such as socio-economic status, education, and community engagement play crucial roles in longevity. Future studies are likely to delve deeper into how these elements interact and how interventions at the community and policy levels can create environments that support healthier, longer lives. For example, urban planning that prioritizes walkability, accessibility to nutritious food, and opportunities for social interaction could have far-reaching impacts on public health.

The potential of wearable technology to monitor and manage health metrics in real-time is also advancing rapidly. Devices that track everything from heart rate variability to sleep quality are becoming increasingly sophisticated. The data collected by these wearables can offer actionable insights, empowering individuals to make informed decisions about their health. As these devices become more integrated into our daily lives, they will likely play a significant role in both preventative healthcare and longevity promotion.

Lastly, the emerging field of epigenetics offers a fascinating glimpse into how our environment and behaviors can influence gene expression and, consequently, aging. Epigenetic changes are reversible modifications to our DNA that do not alter the genetic code but can affect how genes are turned on or off. Factors such as diet, stress, and exposure to toxins can all induce epigenetic changes. Understanding these mechanisms opens up possibilities for interventions that could delay aging and extend lifespan by promoting positive epigenetic modifications while mitigating negative ones.

As we look toward the future, it's clear that the field of longevity science is poised for transformative growth. While the quest for immortality may be as old as humanity itself, today's research and technological advancements bring us closer than ever to truly enhancing both the quantity and quality of life. The journey is ongoing, but each new discovery sheds light on the complex puzzle of aging, bringing hope and inspiration to all who aspire to live healthier, longer lives.

In the end, the most promising aspect of these scientific advancements is how they empower us to take control of our aging process. Whether through adopting healthier lifestyles, leveraging new technologies, or participating in clinical research, each step forward is a step towards a future where longevity is not merely about surviving but thriving. The future is bright, and it holds the potential to transform how we live, age, and experience the world around us. So, as we continue to explore this fascinating field, let's embrace the possibilities it offers and commit to a journey towards a longer, healthier life.

Chapter 12:
Transforming Your Life

Transforming your life is an ongoing journey that requires both commitment and courage, but the rewards—improved health, increased longevity, and enhanced well-being—are immeasurable. Start by incorporating small, actionable tips into your daily routine like those we've discussed in earlier chapters. Picture your life as a blueprint for health; assess areas that need change and gradually evolve them. Real-life success stories show that it's possible to make these shifts. Whether it's adopting a plant-based diet, prioritizing regular physical activity, or finding purpose and meaning, remember that every step counts. Your transformation doesn't have to happen overnight; it's about making consistent, meaningful choices that align with a healthy and fulfilling life. This chapter is your guide to unearthing the tools and inspiration you need to create lasting change, set realistic goals, and build a happier, healthier future—starting now.

Actionable Tips for Longevity

In this transformative journey toward enhanced longevity and well-being, actionable steps become the linchpin to turning aspirations into reality. Building upon evidence derived from the fascinating Blue Zones, integrating longevity practices into your daily life doesn't require a complete overhaul but rather thoughtful, incremental changes. Let's dive into some actionable tips that can set you on the path to a healthier, longer life.

First and foremost, one of the easiest yet most impactful changes you can make is to incorporate plant-based foods into your diet. Research consistently shows that diets rich in vegetables, fruits, legumes, and whole grains are linked to longevity. You don't need to become a vegan overnight. Start by adding an extra serving of vegetables to your lunch and dinner. Over time, these small changes can add up, significantly boosting your nutrient intake and overall health.

Physical activity is a cornerstone of longevity, but it's not about hitting the gym for an hour every day. The key is to move naturally throughout your day. You can start by making simple changes such as taking the stairs instead of the elevator, walking or biking for your errands, or even incorporating stretches and light exercises during TV commercial breaks. The goal is to make movement a seamless part of your daily routine, rather than something that feels like a chore.

Equally important is finding your purpose or Ikigai, as it's called in Okinawa. This sense of purpose can be a powerful motivator that drives you to get out of bed each morning. Reflect on what makes you come alive, what you're good at, and where you feel you can make a positive contribution. Whether it's through your profession, hobbies, or volunteer activities, having a clear sense of purpose can add years to your life by infusing your days with meaning and direction.

Social connections are another crucial element. Foster relationships with family, friends, and your community. Loneliness has been shown to have a comparable impact on health as smoking or obesity. Make a point to reconnect with an old friend, join a club or group that interests you, or simply spend more time with loved ones. The quality of your relationships can significantly influence your longevity, providing emotional support and enhancing your mental and physical well-being.

Managing stress is paramount. Chronic stress not only deteriorates mental health but also has profound effects on physical health, accelerating the aging process. Develop daily relaxation techniques such as deep breathing, meditation, or yoga. Establishing a routine for downtime will help you carve out moments of peace amidst the hustle and bustle of daily life. Even just a few minutes a day dedicated to relaxation can make a substantial difference.

Creating a healthy living environment is another essential step. Your surroundings can greatly influence your lifestyle choices. Aim to design a home that encourages healthy habits. Place fruits and vegetables on your kitchen counter, make your dining area a no-screen zone, and position exercise equipment within easy reach. These small changes can subtly guide you towards healthier behaviors without requiring constant willpower.

Faith and spirituality can also play a significant role in enhancing longevity. Engaging in spiritual practices, whether it's attending religious services, meditating, or simply spending time in nature, can provide a sense of peace and belonging. These activities help you connect with something greater than yourself, providing comfort and reducing stress, which plays a critical role in longevity.

Quality sleep is non-negotiable. Prioritize creating a restful environment conducive to good sleep. This includes maintaining a consistent sleep schedule, limiting screen time before bed, and ensuring your bedroom is dark, quiet, and cool. Good sleep not only rejuvenates your body but also supports cognitive function and emotional health, critical components of a long, healthy life.

Establishing healthy habits is fundamental. These can include simple but powerful practices like staying hydrated, practicing gratitude, and setting aside time for self-care. Avoid harmful behaviors like smoking and excessive alcohol consumption. Instead, focus on positive daily practices that contribute to your overall well-being. The key is consistency; small actions performed daily have a cumulative effect that can significantly impact your longevity.

Lastly, keep informed with scientific insights. Stay updated on new research and findings in the field of longevity. Knowledge empowers you to make informed decisions about your health. Follow credible sources, and if possible, consult with healthcare professionals who can provide personalized advice based on the latest scientific evidence.

Embrace these actionable tips as a holistic approach to enhancing your longevity. Remember, it's not about making drastic changes overnight but about consistent, small steps that align with the principles observed in the world's Blue Zones. Each tip is a piece of the puzzle, contributing to a comprehensive blueprint for a healthier, longer life. This journey is uniquely yours; take each step mindfully, knowing that every positive change brings you closer to unlocking the secrets of longevity.

Real-Life Success Stories

Transforming your life isn't just a theoretical possibility; it's a lived reality for countless individuals around the world. Meet Lisa, a 58-year-old grandmother of three, whose life took a transformational turn after she adopted lifestyle changes inspired by Blue Zones. Lisa was struggling with multiple health issues, including high blood pressure and chronic fatigue, which severely affected her quality of life. However, she was determined to find a way to enjoy her golden years with her grandchildren.

After learning about Blue Zones, Lisa decided to overhaul her diet and incorporate more plant-based foods. She joined a local community garden program, where she not only grew her own vegetables but also made new friends. Over time, her energy levels surged, and her blood pressure normalized. Just last week, she completed a 5K run, something she never thought possible a few years back.

Then there's Thomas, a 65-year-old retiree who struggled with feelings of isolation after the passing of his wife. For Thomas, the social structures and support networks characteristic of Blue Zones communities became a lifeline. He started attending a weekly group that focused on shared hobbies, whether it was gardening, cooking, or even dancing. These gatherings provided him not only with companionship but also with a renewed sense of purpose. Today, Thomas leads the group and inspires others with his resilience and zest for life.

Another remarkable story is that of Maria, a 70-year-old artist from Sardinia—one of the original Blue Zones. Maria had always been passionate about her craft but found it increasingly difficult to maintain her physical and mental well-being as she aged. When she embraced the concept of moving naturally, everything changed. Instead of going to the gym, she made a habit of walking to art classes and carrying her own supplies. The act of integrating physical activity into her daily routines allowed Maria to stay fit without it feeling like a chore. Not only did her physical health improve, but her creativity also soared.

Then we have Raj, a tech executive who faced burnout due to the high demands of his job. Raj's transformation began with simple stress reduction techniques—meditation, mindful breathing, and taking short breaks throughout the day. At first, it felt nearly impossible to carve out time for these practices, but as he persisted, he noticed substantial improvements in his focus and overall well-being. Raj's experience serves as a testament to the power of small, consistent changes that can counteract even the most stressful environments.

Jessica, a middle-aged mom from California, decided to transform her life after reading about the power of purpose and meaning in longevity. She realized that her life had become a monotonous routine of work and family commitments, leaving her feeling uninspired and drained. By identifying her "Ikigai"—a Japanese concept that translates to "reason for being"—she rekindled her passion for writing. Jessica began setting aside just 15 minutes each day to write, and this small act infused her life with newfound joy and satisfaction. Now, she writes a blog that has a growing readership, inspiring others to find their own purpose.

Let's not overlook Manuel, a 75-year-old farmer from Costa Rica's Nicoya Peninsula, another famed Blue Zone. Manuel attributes his longevity to his lifestyle of natural movement and simple living. From tending to his crops to walking to the nearby village for social outings, Manuel's daily activities are imbued with purpose and physical engagement. His diet, rich in beans, rice, and fresh fruits, complements his active lifestyle. Manuel's story serves as a powerful reminder that sometimes, the simplest changes yield the most significant results.

Meghan, a young professional, found her transformation through faith and spirituality. She often found herself overwhelmed by the rapid pace of modern life and sought a way to ground herself. By incorporating spiritual practices such as yoga and meditation into her daily routine, she found a sense of inner peace and stability. Meghan now experiences less anxiety and has improved focus, which has translated into better performance at work and more meaningful connections with her loved ones.

Even children have not been left untouched by these transformative practices. Take the example of 10-year-old Leo, whose family adopted a Blue Zone-inspired lifestyle to improve their collective well-being. His parents replaced their usual fast food dinners with home-cooked, plant-based meals, and encouraged more outdoor play. The changes worked wonders for Leo's health; he now has more energy, improved grades, and a more radiant outlook on life. This family transformation story showcases how longevity practices can benefit all ages.

Another life changed is that of Samuel, who was diagnosed with Type 2 diabetes. Inspired by Blue Zones, Samuel swapped his sedentary lifestyle for one full of natural movement. He began biking to work, opting for stairs over elevators, and gardening. His diet also shifted to more nutrient-dense foods. Just ten months later, Samuel's doctors were astonished by his progress; his blood sugar levels were under control, and he had lost weight without feeling deprived.

Finally, we have Hanna, a 45-year-old businesswoman, who struggled with sleep issues for years. Hanna's transformation came from embracing Blue Zone sleep practices. She created a restful environment by eliminating electronics from her bedroom and adopting a consistent sleep schedule. Her sleep quality and overall health improved drastically. Now, Hanna feels refreshed every morning, ready to tackle her day with zest and positivity.

These real-life success stories exemplify how individuals from various walks of life have embraced the principles of Blue Zones to transform their lives. The key takeaway from these stories is that change is indeed possible, regardless of age or current circumstances. The common thread among these individuals is their unwavering commitment to making consistent, small adjustments that collectively make a big difference. Whether it's through changes in diet, increased physical activity, building community connections, or finding purpose, these changes are accessible and attainable. And most importantly, they offer a roadmap to a healthier and more fulfilling life.

Every journey is unique, and everyone's starting point is different. What these stories illustrate is the transformative power of taking that first step. Harness the lessons from these real-life success stories to guide your journey towards a healthier and longer life. Remember, you're not just adding years to life but life to your years.

Developing Your Blueprint for a Healthy Life

In our journey towards a healthier life, a solid plan acts as your compass. With the right blueprint, you don't just live; you thrive. When it comes to enhancing longevity, the principles we've talked about intersect and symbiotically reinforce one another, guiding you to a life that's not just longer but richer and more meaningful. But how do we put these myriad principles into a cohesive plan? Let's break it down.

Firstly, identify your starting point. Take stock of where you are today, both physically and mentally. What are your eating habits? How active are you? How connected do you feel to your community and your sense of purpose? Knowing your current state helps you identify areas for improvement and sets a baseline for measuring progress. It may seem daunting, but reflection is your first step towards transformation.

Once you have a clear sense of your starting point, it's time to visualize where you want to go. Define your vision of a healthy life. Visualizations can be immensely powerful. Do you see yourself more physically active, eating cleaner, or perhaps feeling more at peace? Your vision acts like a beacon, guiding each decision and action. Make sure this vision is vivid and inspiring; it should compel you to take action each day.

Next, let's outline small, actionable steps to bring that vision to life. Grand changes often start with small steps. If diet is an area of focus, consider incorporating more plant-based meals. Start with Meatless Mondays or try adding a new vegetable to your dinner plate each week. Simplify your goals into tiny, manageable tasks that bring immediate, though incremental, benefits. This not only makes the process less intimidating but also helps build momentum.

Speaking of momentum, it's essential to establish routines. Habits are life's autopilot. By incorporating healthy habits into your daily routine, you create a stable foundation. Try dedicating 20 minutes each morning to a physical activity you enjoy. Whether it's yoga, a brisk walk, or a quick session of jumping jacks, consistency is key. Repeating these activities solidifies them as part of your lifestyle, eventually becoming second nature.

However, life is anything but linear. You'll face setbacks and obstacles. Stress, temptation, and life's unpredictabilities will test your resolve. Prepare for these moments by developing resilience—both mentally and physically. Embrace stress-reduction techniques that work for you. Deep breathing, mindfulness, or even a short walk can recalibrate your mind and body. This journey isn't about perfection; it's about progress and adaptability.

Moreover, don't underestimate the power of your environment. Surround yourself with cues that remind you of your goals. A bowl of fresh fruits on your kitchen table can act as a visual prompt to eat healthier. Limit junk food in your pantry to reduce temptation. Simple changes to your surroundings can have a profound impact on your behavior.

Community support is another cornerstone of your blueprint. Humans are social creatures and your environment includes your social circle. Surround yourself with people who inspire and support your journey. Share your goals with family and friends. Join a community group or a class where you can meet like-minded individuals. Social bonds not only keep you accountable but also enhance your emotional well-being.

Let's also talk about the role of purpose. Your ikigai, or reason for being, isn't just a philosophical concept; it's a practical tool for living a longer, more fulfilling life. Take time to discover what fuels your passion. This could be a hobby, a volunteer activity, or even a personal project that brings you joy. Purpose ties your blueprint together, providing meaning to your daily actions and long-term goals.

Tracking your progress is vital. A journal or a dedicated app to log daily activities, dietary choices, and emotional states can be incredibly helpful. It allows you to see patterns, identify what works, and pinpoint areas needing adjustment. Regularly reviewing these logs provides a sense of accomplishment and keeps you motivated.

There's also the matter of flexibility. Your blueprint isn't set in stone. Be open to changes and ready to adapt. Life shifts, and so should your plans. If a particular approach isn't working for you, don't be afraid to adjust it. Flexibility ensures that your journey remains sustainable and tailored to your evolving needs and circumstances.

Being kind to yourself throughout this process is essential. Self-compassion helps maintain a positive mindset and keeps you motivated even when progress seems slow. Celebrate small victories and don't dwell on setbacks. Remember, this journey is about building a healthier and more fulfilling life, not adhering to rigid rules.

Regularly revisiting and updating your blueprint also serves to keep it relevant. As you progress, your needs and goals will evolve. Every few months, reflect and adjust your plan to make sure it aligns with your current state and future aspirations. This continuous refinement keeps the journey dynamic and engaging.

Finally, remember that you're not alone. The principles and practices discussed throughout this book have been tested and proven by communities that have thrived for centuries. You have the wisdom of these collective experiences to guide and inspire you. Look to these examples for encouragement and proof that transforming your life through evidence-based, healthy changes is entirely achievable.

To sum up, developing your blueprint for a healthy life involves a multi-layered approach. It starts with honest self-assessment and visualization, blossoms through small, actionable steps, and is fortified by community support, purpose, and flexibility. Continuously tracking progress and revisiting your blueprint ensures it remains a living document, adapting to guide you towards a longer, healthier, and more joyful life. This is your masterpiece in the making, one brushstroke at a time.

So take that first step. Start with a plan, no matter how simple. It's the small changes, compounded over time, that yield the most remarkable transformations. Here's to your journey towards crafting a life that's not just longer but infinitely richer in meaning and joy.

Conclusion

As we reach the end of our journey into the myriad facets that contribute to a long, healthy life, it's crucial to reflect on the wisdom that our exploration of Blue Zones has provided. These regions, with their exceptional longevity blessings, offer a treasure trove of insights applicable to all of us, no matter where we reside. The ultimate goal is clear: to empower, inspire, and instruct you to integrate these practices into your daily life for better long-term health and wellbeing.

Adopting the habits observed in Blue Zones isn't merely about adding years to your life; it's about adding life to your years. This means embracing a lifestyle that enhances your physical health, mental peace, and emotional wellbeing. From forging strong communal bonds to enjoying a plant-based diet abundant in natural flavors and nutrients, each section of this book has offered practical steps to cultivate habits conducive to longevity.

But these changes don't need to be monumental overnight transformations. Start small. Incorporate more vegetables into your diet, take a daily walk, or make it a point to call a loved one more often. Each of these incremental changes builds a foundation for a healthier life. Over time, they create a cumulative, positive impact that can be profoundly transformative.

It's essential to emphasize that living longer and healthier isn't limited by geography. While the specific practices of Blue Zones are derived from their unique cultures, the underlying principles are universal. The power of community, the need for purposeful living, the importance of stress reduction, and the beauty of simplicity are concepts that transcend borders. They are applicable in any context and can be adapted to fit your personal circumstances.

Of course, science plays a critical role in substantiating these practices. Rigorous research validates that the habits found in Blue Zones are not mere folklore but powerful elements that contribute to remarkable longevity. By marrying anecdotal wisdom with scientific inquiry, we ensure that the recommendations provided here stand on a solid foundation of evidence and practical applicability.

Think of your journey to longevity as crafting a masterpiece. Each brushstroke adds detail and depth, culminating in something beautiful and enduring. There's no rush. Take your time to paint your life with the colors of healthy habits, supportive relationships, purposeful actions, and joyful moments.

We must also recognize the importance of adaptability. As life's circumstances change, so too should your approach to these longevity practices. Be flexible. Allow yourself the grace to adjust your routines and practices as needed. What's important is not perfection, but consistency and commitment to a healthier lifestyle.

And let's not forget about joy and fulfillment. Longevity is as much about happiness as it is about health. Engage in activities that bring you joy, nurture your passions, and enrich your spirit. Whether it's gardening, cooking with loved ones, volunteering, or simply spending time in nature, find what makes your heart sing and make it a regular part of your life.

In closing, take a moment to envision what a longer, healthier life looks like for you. Picture the energy, vitality, and peace you'll gain. Visualize the stronger relationships you'll build, the dreams you'll pursue, and the legacy of health and happiness you'll leave behind. This vision is not a distant fantasy. With dedication to the principles outlined in this book, it's a reality within your reach.

Your longevity journey begins now. Each step you take, no matter how small, is a declaration of your commitment to a vibrant, fulfilling life. Here's to your health, your happiness, and your many years ahead.

Thank you for embarking on this transformative journey. May it be the start of a life filled with vitality, purpose, and profound wellbeing.

Appendix A:
Appendix

This appendix serves as an invaluable resource to help you fully embrace the longevity practices discussed throughout this book. Here, you'll find a curated selection of recipes from Blue Zones that capture the essence of a diet rich in plant-based foods, delightfully simple yet nutritionally robust. Additionally, a comprehensive list of resources for further reading will enable you to dive deeper into the science and traditions that underpin these healthy lifestyles, broadening your understanding and inspiring continued growth. Finally, a meticulously crafted checklist for longevity practices will guide you in systematically integrating these transformative habits into your daily life, empowering you to enhance your well-being and extend your lifespan. This section is designed to be your go-to reference, offering practical tools and inspiration to support your journey towards a healthier, more vibrant life.

Recipes from Blue Zones

Exploring culinary traditions from Blue Zones allows us a glimpse into the simplicity and richness of diets that have nurtured some of the world's longest-living populations. The culinary secrets from these regions aren't mysterious potions but simple, wholesome ingredients combined thoughtfully to enhance both flavor and nutrition. Rooted deeply in their cultures and lifestyles, these recipes offer a roadmap to longevity that embraces the idea of 'food as medicine.'

Let's begin our journey in Okinawa, Japan, where the diet is rich in vegetables, tofu, fish, and small amounts of pork. One staple dish is the Okinawan sweet potato, or *satsuma-imo*. It's a vibrant purple tuber packed with antioxidants and dietary fiber. A popular way to prepare it is by simply steaming or roasting, then lightly garnishing with a sprinkle of sea salt, allowing its natural sweetness to shine.

Another Okinawan staple is *goya champuru*, a stir-fry featuring bitter melon, tofu, and sometimes a bit of pork or egg. The bitterness of the goya requires an acquired taste, but it's believed to boost metabolism and help stabilize blood sugar levels. A typical recipe might include sautéing sliced bitter melon with firm tofu, onions, and a light soy sauce dressing, offering not just a meal but a symphony of textures and flavors that dance on your palate.

Moving to Ikaria, Greece, a Blue Zone known for its Mediterranean diet, we find a plethora of inspiration. One revered dish is *fasolada*, a traditional Greek bean soup. This hearty dish includes simple ingredients such as white beans, tomatoes, carrots, celery, onions, and olive oil. Seasoned with bay leaves and thyme, fasolada embodies the Ikarian focus on legumes and vegetables, providing a comforting, nutritionally dense meal.

Ikarians also enjoy foraged greens known as *horta*. These wild greens, often dandelion or amaranth, are boiled and served with a drizzle of olive oil and fresh lemon juice. The inherent bitterness of these greens signifies their abundant phytonutrients, believed to combat inflammation and promote heart health.

Sardinia, Italy, another Blue Zone, offers its own culinary treasures, particularly through its emphasis on whole grains, beans, and vegetables. The Sardinian diet includes a focus on barley, often featured in the regional dish *migliarisu* – a barley soup with vegetables and sometimes a touch of pecorino cheese. This dish is a reminder of the nutritional power of whole grains, providing a hefty serving of fiber, vitamins, and minerals without complicated preparation.

Additionally, Sardinia is known for *minestrone*, a vegetable soup that showcases a variety of garden-fresh produce, beans, and pasta. Each bowl of minestrone not only warms the body but also fortifies it with vital nutrients. Sardinians often prepare this soup in large batches, appreciating the convenience of having multiple nutritious meals ready to go.

Costa Rica's Nicoya Peninsula is a Blue Zone where corn, beans, and squash – the "three sisters" – form the dietary staples. A quintessential Nicoyan recipe is *gallo pinto*, a flavorful combination of black beans and rice. Prepared with a medley of onions, bell peppers, cilantro, and sometimes a dash of *Salsa Lizano*, gallo pinto is not only filling but also provides a perfect balance of protein and complex carbohydrates.

Another Nicoyan favorite is *chorreadas*, corn pancakes made from fresh corn kernels. Blended into a batter with a bit of salt and water, then cooked on a hot griddle, chorreadas are often enjoyed with a smear of fresh cheese or a dollop of sour cream. The simplicity and natural sweetness of fresh corn make this dish a delightful, nutrient-packed treat.

In Loma Linda, California, home to one of the highest concentrations of Seventh-day Adventists, the diet aligns closely with the plant-based principles seen in other Blue Zones. A cherished recipe from this community is the hearty *Adventist lentil stew*. This satisfying stew features lentils, carrots, potatoes, and an assortment of spices, simmered to perfection. The result is a nutrient-dense meal rich in plant-based protein, fiber, and essential micronutrients like iron and folate.

Adventists also enjoy a variety of homemade nut-based milks and butters, reflecting their focus on natural, minimally processed foods.

Almond milk, made by blending soaked almonds with water and straining, provides a nutritious alternative to dairy, replete with vitamins E and D.

As we consider adopting these recipes into our own culinary repertoire, it's important to remember that the beauty of Blue Zone cooking lies in its simplicity. Many of these dishes come together with minimal ingredients and straightforward techniques, making them accessible even to those who might not consider themselves culinary aficionados.

By embracing the ethos of these Blue Zones – prioritizing whole, nutrient-rich foods prepared with care – we're not just cooking meals but creating a lifestyle. Our choices at the grocery store and in the kitchen become acts of self-care, aligning us with the habits of some of the world's longest-lived people. We're reminded that great health doesn't arise from fleeting diet trends but from sustained, thoughtful choices made day after day.

As we journey further into the secrets of longevity, these recipes serve as both inspiration and practical tools. They teach us to appreciate the bounty of the earth, to revel in the simplicity of fresh, wholesome ingredients, and to enjoy the process of creating meals that nourish both body and soul. By weaving these culinary traditions into our lives, we take a crucial step toward not just living longer, but living better.

Resources for Further Reading

The vast and complex journey towards enhancing longevity and quality of life is made easier with the right resources. While this book provides a comprehensive introduction to the practices that promote longevity, further exploration is vital for deepening your understanding. Below, I've curated a selection of insightful books, influential studies, and valuable online resources that will amplify your knowledge and inspire actionable change.

First, let's turn to books authored by experts in the fields of nutrition, wellness, and longevity. Consider reading "How Not to Die" by Dr. Michael Greger. This book delves into the role of diet in preventing disease and promoting longevity. Dr. Greger's meticulous review of scientific evidence provides compelling arguments for adopting a plant-based diet, echoing some of the key dietary principles found in Blue Zones.

Another essential read is "The Blue Zones Solution" by Dan Buettner. This book is more than just a follow-up to his initial exploration of Blue Zones; it's a practical guide that offers specific strategies and recipes inspired by the longevity hotspots around the world. Buettner's work beautifully combines storytelling with actionable insights, making it an engaging and educational resource.

If you're looking for something that intersects well with stress management and purpose, "Man's Search for Meaning" by Viktor Frankl is indispensable. Frankl's exploration of finding purpose amidst life's greatest challenges resonates deeply with the concept of 'ikigai,' a foundational element in achieving a longer, meaningful life. His perspective on the psychological aspects of resilience and purpose complements the more tactical advice found elsewhere.

In addition to these books, scientific literature provides a treasure trove of information on longevity. Peer-reviewed journals such as "The Lancet" and "JAMA" (Journal of the American Medical Association) frequently publish groundbreaking studies on nutrition, exercise, and chronic disease management. Seeking out these primary sources can give you a more nuanced understanding of the evidence underlying longevity practices.

For those who prefer interactive and multidisciplinary exploring, online courses can be a substantial resource. Platforms like Coursera and EdX offer courses from top universities that cover topics such as nutrition, exercise physiology, and behavioral science. The "Science of

Well-Being" course offered by Yale University is particularly popular. It provides practical, research-backed strategies for improving your happiness and well-being, which are intrinsically linked to longevity.

Websites and blogs by well-regarded experts also serve as up-to-the-minute resources on longevity. Websites like NutritionFacts.org, maintained by Dr. Michael Greger, provide video breakdowns of the latest nutrition research, while blogs by experts like Mark Hyman, MD, offer insights into functional medicine and holistic wellness.

Subscribing to newsletters from longevity-focused organizations can also keep you informed. The American College of Lifestyle Medicine (ACLM) often shares latest research findings and practical advice for integrating lifestyle changes into your daily routine.

Documentaries are another accessible and impactful way to enhance your knowledge. For instance, "Forks Over Knives" explores the transformative power of plant-based diets. "Awake: The Life of Yogananda" delves into the spiritual aspects of well-being, echoing the emphasis on faith and spirituality for longevity found in Blue Zones.

Moreover, podcasts offer a convenient way to absorb information on the go. "The Doctor's Farmacy" with Dr. Mark Hyman often features discussions with leading experts in nutrition, functional medicine, and wellness. Similarly, "Rich Roll Podcast" frequently includes episodes focused on health, fitness, and longevity, featuring inspiring stories from individuals who have transformed their lives.

In this digital age, social media platforms also act as dynamic resources. Following credible experts on Twitter, Instagram, or LinkedIn can provide daily motivation and tips. Look for accounts that share peer-reviewed research, personal stories of transformation, and practical advice grounded in science.

To deeply explore Blue Zones diets and recipes, consider digital cooking classes and platforms like MasterClass. Classes led by renowned chefs who focus on plant-based cooking can transform your kitchen into a mini Blue Zone, helping you integrate these longevity-promoting meals into your daily routine.

For a community-based approach, join local wellness groups or online forums focused on longevity. Websites like Meetup.com list various groups where you can participate in book discussions, attend wellness workshops, or join social gatherings that promote healthy living.

Lastly, don't underestimate the power of self-experimentation combined with mindfulness. Keeping a personal journal of your habits, diet, exercise, and stress levels can be enlightening. Reflecting on what you've read and observed will help integrate new practices into your life more seamlessly. By noting changes and patterns, you can tailor your longevity practices to what works best for you personally.

While this book lays a strong foundation, these additional resources can provide a wealth of knowledge and inspiration. Through continuous learning and application, you'll be well-equipped to cultivate a lifestyle that not only enhances your longevity but also enriches your overall quality of life. Dive into these resources, keep an open mind, and remain committed to lifelong wellness. The journey to a healthier, longer life is as enriching as the destination itself.

Checklist for Longevity Practices

To ensure that you're on the right track towards living a long and fulfilling life, here's a comprehensive checklist to guide you. This checklist incorporates the evidence-based practices from the world's Blue Zones, where people live the longest and healthiest lives. Follow these guidelines consistently, and you'll find yourself on a path to better health and greater longevity.

1. **Adopt a Plant-Based Diet:**

Focusing on whole, plant-based foods such as fruits, vegetables, legumes, nuts, and whole grains can significantly benefit your health. Limit meat consumption and consider adopting a Mediterranean or a more plant-focused diet, as they are commonly associated with greater longevity.

2. **Embrace Natural Movement:**

Engage in regular physical activity that mimics the natural movements found in everyday tasks. This can include walking, gardening, and manual labor. The key is to stay active without necessarily hitting the gym. Find ways to incorporate movement into your daily life, like taking the stairs instead of the elevator or biking to work.

3. **Stay Connected**

Build and maintain strong social relationships. Investing in family and friendships can offer emotional and psychological support, which are critical components of longevity. Make time for social gatherings, and don't hesitate to reach out to loved ones regularly.

4. **Find Your Purpose**

Having a sense of purpose can add years to your life. Identify what drives you, and make it a focal point of your daily activities. Whether it's a career, a hobby, volunteering, or family responsibilities, having a "why" for getting out of bed in the morning is crucial.

5. **Reduce Stress**

Chronic stress is a major deterrent to longevity. Implement daily relaxation techniques such as yoga, meditation, or simple breathing exercises. Make room for downtime in your schedule, and don't shy away from activities that bring you joy and relaxation.

6. Prioritize Restful Sleep:

Healthy sleep habits are essential for physical and mental well-being. Aim for 7-8 hours of quality sleep each night. Create a restful sleep environment by keeping your bedroom cool, dark, and quiet. Avoid electronics before bedtime to enhance your sleep quality.

7. Engage in Spiritual Practices:

Whether through organized religion or personal spirituality, engaging in spiritual practices can enhance your sense of belonging and purpose. This can be as simple as taking a few moments for gratitude every day or participating in a faith community.

8. Design Your Environment:

Surround yourself with a longevity-promoting environment. This includes living spaces that encourage physical activity and community interaction. Design your home and workspace to promote movement, healthy eating, and socialization. The right environment reduces the need for willpower and makes healthy choices the default option.

9. Establish Healthy Habits:

Form habits that promote health and longevity. Small, positive changes can accumulate over time to significantly impact your well-being. Whether it's a daily walk, a balanced breakfast, or setting aside time to read, these habits can lead to a healthier, more fulfilling life.

10. Moderate Alcohol Consumption:

If you drink alcohol, do so in moderation. This often means a glass of red wine with meals, which can be part of a social and balanced lifestyle. Excessive drinking can have detrimental effects on your health, so finding a balance is key.

11. Engage in Lifelong Learning:

Keep your brain active through continuous learning and mental challenges. Read, solve puzzles, learn new skills, or engage in intellectually stimulating conversations. Intellectual engagement is a significant factor in healthy aging and longevity.

12. Limit Harmful Behaviors:

Avoid behaviors that negatively impact your health, such as smoking, excessive drinking, and a sedentary lifestyle. These not only shorten your lifespan but also diminish the quality of the years you do have.

13. Pursue Meaningful Leisure Activities:

Engage in hobbies and activities that bring you joy and fulfillment. Whether it's painting, fishing, dancing, or any other leisure activity, make time for the things you love. These activities contribute to your overall happiness and well-being.

14. Stay Hydrated:

Drink plenty of water throughout the day. Staying hydrated is essential for maintaining bodily functions and overall health. Aim for at least 8 glasses a day, and adjust based on your activity level and climate conditions.

15. Practice Gratitude:

Regularly take time to reflect on what you're thankful for. Practicing gratitude can enhance your emotional health, reduce stress, and increase your overall sense of well-being. This simple act can have profound effects on your mindset and longevity.

16. Eat in Moderation:

Practice mindful eating and listen to your body's hunger cues. Instead of overeating, aim for a balanced diet that nourishes you without excess. Mindful eating helps you enjoy your meals more while promoting a healthy weight.

17. Consider Periodic Fasting:

Intermittent fasting or periods of reduced calorie intake have been associated with longevity. Always consult with a healthcare provider before starting any fasting regimen to ensure it's safe for your individual health needs.

18. Access Reliable Health Information:

Stay informed about your health by accessing reliable sources of information. Seek guidance from healthcare professionals, and keep up with the latest research on longevity. An informed approach to health allows you to make better choices.

19. Embrace Optimism:

A positive outlook on life can significantly impact your longevity. Embrace optimism and work on developing a resilient mindset. Focus on the good, practice forgiveness, and cultivate an attitude of growth and possibility.

This checklist, while comprehensive, is just a starting point. Everyone's journey to longevity is unique, and it's essential to tailor these practices to fit your individual lifestyle and needs. By incorporating these evidence-based practices, you're creating a foundation for a longer, healthier, and more fulfilling life. Remember, consistency is key. Small changes, made regularly, can lead to profound and lasting results.

Now, armed with these guidelines, take the first